The H PYLORI Diet

The Shocking Truth About Helicobacter Pylori & How You Can Beat Its Symptoms In 60-Days Or Less Without The Need For Antibiotics

May Benefit:

- Heartburn • Stomach Pain • Acid Reflux
- Bloating • Nausea • Excess Gas & Belching
- IBS • Fatigue • Urticaria • Rosacea

David Hompes

Published by
Health For The People Ltd

First published in Great Britain in 2011 by

Health For The People Ltd.
35 Kingsland Road, London, E2 8AA
Tel: 0800 310 21 21
Office@HPExperts.com
www.H-Pylori-Symptoms.com

HEALTH DISCLAIMER
The information in this book is not intended to diagnose, treat, cure or prevent any disease, nor should it replace a one-to-one relationship with your physician. You should always seek consultation with a qualified medical practitioner before commencing any treatment protocols.

Printed and bound in Great Britain by
CPI Antony Rowe, Chippenham.

British Library Cataloguing in Publication Data.

ISBN 978-0-9569230-0-4

Table of Contents

About The Author...1
Introduction...3
How To Use This Resource 8

Part One – Busting The H Pylori Myths

Introduction to Part One 10

What Is Helicobacter Pylori?..11
Does Everyone Have H Pylori?...12
What Causes H Pylori & Where Does It Come From?........14
Is Stress A Risk Factor For Acquiring H Pylori Infection?...14
Summary & Learning Points...21

How Does H Pylori Get Into Your Body?...........................22

H Pylori, Kissing & Sexual Contact..................................23
Sharing Eating & Drinking Utensils..................................24
Mother to Child & Family Transmission 24
H Pylori in Water 25
H Pylori in Food 26
Hospitals & Endoscopic Procedures.................................26
Pets & Other Animals 26
Yeast Organisms 27
Can I Pass H Pylori To My Children & Loved Ones? 28
Summary 28

What Are The Symptoms of H Pylori?...............................29

Digestive Symptoms Caused By H Pylori 32
Acute Symptoms33
Chronic Symptoms...33
Is H Pylori The Same As Irritable Bowel Syndrome?..........33

Fatigue, Mood, Sleep & Weight Management Problems .34
H Pylori & Skin Disease...36
Can H Pylori Cause Heart Disease.............................38
H Pylori & Stomach Ulcers...43
H Pylori Can Cause Stomach Cancer.......................45
Can H-Pylori Kill?...47

What Tests Are Available For H Pylori?.......................47

What Is The Best Test For H Pylori? 51
Advantages of Comprehensive Stool Testing.......52
Should Your Loved Ones & Family Be Tested?......56
Why Doesn't Your Doctor Tell You All This?.........58

Can H Pylori Be Eradicated? 62

What Is The Best Medical Treatment?.....................64
Patient Screening 67
Side Effects Of H Pylori Treatment 68
H Pylori & Yeast/Fungal Overgrowth 72
Antacids Are Big Business..73
The Nexium 'Scandal'..74
Discontinuing Antacids 78
Final Comment on Antacids.......................................78
Natural Health Alternatives.......................................81
Summary of Part One..82

Part Two - Featuring The H Pylori Diet

Introduction To The H Pylori Diet 83

  No Magic Bullet..84
  Using The H Pylori Diet 85

Understanding Your Digestive System.....................87

  The Three Roles of Your Digestive System.........87
  Digestion from the Top Down...........................88
  The Impact of H Pylori on Your Digestive System 92
  How Does H Pylori Damage Your Stomach?................92
  Gastritis & Ulcers 93
  Secondary Infections 94
  H Pylori and The Gallbladder...........................95

The H Pylori Diet 96

  Take This Programme at Your Own Pace............96
  The Stomach Cleanse 97
  How Quickly Will You See Results? 98

The H Pylori Diet Phase One - Foods To Avoid 99

  Step One - Eliminate Gluten............................99
  Step Two - Eliminate Processed Cow's Milk Foods 106
  Step Three - Avoid Soy 109
  Step Four - Cut Back On Your Sugar Intake..............111
  Step Five - Throw Out The Bad Fats 113
  Phase One - Review.......................................118

Phase Two - Eat More Good Foods 120

  How To Use The H-Pylori Diet Food Guide 120
  Meal/Recipes And Planning Ideas......................127
  Food Quality & Shopping Tips 130

Tips For Busy Lifestyles 133
Healthy Gluten-Free Recipes...138
Supermarket Foods That May Inhibit H Pylori.................151
How To Control Your Blood Sugar Levels 154
How To Optimize Your Digestion.......................................156
How To Eat More Raw Foods Using Vegetable Juicing...158
Water & Hydration Guidelines 163

Phase Three - The Stomach Cleanse...................................169

Timing Of The Stomach Cleanse..170
Best Natural Herbs & Supplements For H Pylori.............171
Which Products & When? 177
How To Order The Stomach Cleanse Products 181
Possible Side Effects & Precautions 181
Stomach Cleanse And Triple Therapy................................182
You Can Make Triple Therapy More Effective 182
Lactoferrin 182
Probiotics 183
General Yeast & Fungal Cleanse & Probiotics..................184
Can Children Use The Stomach Cleanse?.........................186
How Do You Know H Pylori Has Gone? 186
What Is The Best Way of Re-Testing..................................186
Can H Pylori Return? 188
How Can You Stop H Pylori Coming Back?.......................188
What If Symptoms Do Not Go Away? 189
Other Digestive Infections 190
How Long Will It Take Before You Feel Well Again?......192
How Long Should You Follow The Eating Plan? 193
Closing Comments...194

About the Author

Dave Hompes is a Functional Medicine and Clinical Nutrition practitioner based in London, UK. He is regarded as one of the world's leading experts on H pylori. Dave has traveled widely in order to learn his skills from some of the most prominent and successful practitioners in the world.

Having suffered with and overcome H pylori and Blastocystis hominis infections without medical intervention, he spent more than a year researching H pylori so that he could help others overcome the infection and its debilitating symptoms quickly and effectively and has specialised in helping people overcome H pylori using natural methods since 2007.

Dave works out of a clinic in London, UK and maintains an active phone consultation practice, designing nutritional programmes and providing coaching & counseling to improve clients' health through diet and lifestyle modifications. Dave has worked with clients in the UK & Ireland, US and Canada, Holland, Germany, South Africa, the Middle East, Singapore, Australia and New Zealand.

Dave is also a successful author, having written and contributed to several books and publications, including Men's Health Magazine. He has presented at the Royal Society Of Medicine and has made numerous appearances in the press and on the BBC.

Dave's Message

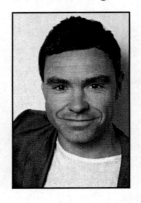

"Having suffered with *H pylori* and *Blastocystis*, I know first-hand how the symptoms caused by these infections can leave you in pain, drain your energy, affect your mood and leave you worried about longer-term consequences such as stomach ulcers and cancer.

It is my experience that some doctors understand the *H pylori* problem relatively well whereas others really do not have the necessary knowledge, skills and experience of the problem to help patients overcome their symptoms. This is particularly the case when conventional antibiotics do not bring relief.

I wrote this guide, which is now in its third edition, so that you can understand the *H pylori* problem in greater detail and utilise the same principles that I used to overcome my H pylori infection quickly and without side effects. It is my hope that you find the information in the following pages helpful and that you are able to overcome your health challenges relatively quickly and inexpensively, as I did."

Wishing you perfect health...

Dave Hompes

Introduction

When I wrote the first e-book edition of *The H Pylori Diet* in 2008, I could scarcely have imagined the response it would generate. Since that time, my Inbox has been bombarded by emails from folk all over the world who have suffered at the hands of *Helicobacter pylori* and its vast array of symptoms and clinical manifestations. My *H pylori* website receives more than one thousand visits each day and our phone lines and email accounts are jammed. All this does is reinforce to me the profound health implications of *H pylori* infection and it drives me to disseminate the information you're about to read to the far flung corners of the Earth.

This project all started, unbeknownst to me, in 2004 when I suffered a nasty bout of food poisoning in Egypt. I lay awake in my hotel room feeling as though someone had shoved a flame-thrower down my throat. I can honestly say that those heartburn and reflux symptoms made me feel like I was going to die – a not too unfamiliar feeling to many *H pylori* suffers. I then spent the night vomiting and the following week on the toilet with diarrhoea. All this was accompanied by nausea and extreme weakness.

Two weeks later, despite returning to the UK, I was still suffering with a combination of anxiety, lethargy, fatigue and a curious white coating on my tongue. In fact, it took well over a month before I actually felt like myself again. As an otherwise sport-mad, fit and healthy personal trainer, whatever that 'thing' was, it really knocked me out. However, despite all those symptoms and purely through personal choice, I did not actually visit a doctor.

Fast forwarding to September 2007, I'd made some decisions in my business and personal life that proved to be, let's say, "less than optimal". Basically, I lost a lot of money in a business venture that didn't go very well and ended up socialising heavily to escape the precarious financial situation

3

I'd landed myself in. In fact, on February 21st, 2007, I had to declare myself bankrupt at the High Court of Justice on London's Strand. The weeks and months leading up to this event were incredibly stressful and those flame-thrower heartburn and reflux symptoms returned with a vengeance. As before, they were accompanied by fatigue and anxiety. I was also having a hard time sleeping and, oddly, sustaining an erection.

As you might imagine, as a fit and healthy personal trainer it doesn't look very good to your clients if you're feeling tired and ill all the time! Despite eating a very healthy diet and exercising appropriately, I couldn't get myself to feel better. Fortunately, in April 2007, I began a six-month course in "Functional Medicine". I was studying with Dr. Dan Kalish, a fifteen-year veteran of Functional Medicine in California.

Functional medicine is a discipline that's gaining significant momentum in North America, but not so much in the UK, Europe, Australasia and other parts of the world. The core premise of functional medicine is that health can be regained and maintained through optimal nutrition and lifestyle habits. On top of this foundation, functional laboratory assessments can then be used to identify imbalances in the key systems of the body. These key systems can then be rebalanced and, as a result, the majority of symptoms and even what we have come to know as "diseases" can often be resolved.

Functional medicine was my saviour. As part of my education I was required to submit a stool sample (with a private laboratory in California), that was analysed for bacteria, parasites and fungal overgrowth. Lo and behold, my test result came back positive for *H pylori*. This clearly explained my digestive symptoms. I also ran a saliva test that checked the balance of my stress hormones, namely cortisol and DHEA. My cortisol levels were completely "upside down". At 8am they were too low and at 11pm they were way too high. I realised that the intense stress I had been under as a result of my financial situation had contributed significantly to the imbalances and that the findings went a long way to explaining why I wasn't sleeping well and why my energy levels were so erratic.

Because I generally avoid taking any form of medical drug unless it is completely necessary, I chose to pursue a natural approach to help resolve my symptoms. Dr. Kalish provided me a 'stomach cleanse' that would work against the *H pylori* and also a hormone-boosting protocol to help with energy levels and sleep. Within 90-days, 85% of my symptoms had cleared up and I literally felt like a new man. When I ran a re-test, there was no longer any sign of *H pylori*. Some other interesting bugs did show up, including a parasite and some fungal overgrowth. These are discussed later in the book.

I was astonished at how quickly some simple tests and recommendations had helped me recover and felt compelled to find a way to share the information with as many people as possible. I decided to research *H pylori*, set up a simple website with some free information and run phone consultations to help folk understand the problem in more depth. Within just a few days of advertising the website on Google, I began receiving emails from confused people who didn't really know where to turn with their symptoms.

The rest is history, so they say, and this book is the culmination of the last three year's research and diligent work with many hundreds of individuals around the world who were previously unable to resolve their *H pylori* infections, associated symptoms and health challenges. I'm pleased to say that the majority of these people have been able to overcome their symptoms and return to normal, vibrant health.

Through my hands-on work with clients and through the letters and emails we receive on a daily basis, it has become clear to me that the medical system is not doing a very good job of helping people with *H pylori* and the acute and chronic symptoms that accompany its presence.

I've identified five major problems with *H pylori*:

1. A lot of people have it and, contrary to what most doctors believe, it *can* be passed from person-to-person.

2. A lot of people don't even realise they have it. Instead, they walk around complaining that they're struggling with symptoms that they believe are normal because most of their friends also have the same symptoms!

3. A lot of doctors are reluctant to run testing because they feel it is too expensive and, depending on which country we're talking about, their budgets don't allow it.

4. Even when testing is performed, it's not always accurate and they don't test for the right things!

5. Even when diagnosis of *H pylori* is confirmed, the treatments are not always effective and can actually make people feel worse.

The good news is that *H pylori* is not only manageable, it's completely curable. But in order for success to be achieved, it's *essential* to get the facts right and understand the problems and challenges in a little more detail, which is why you and I are together with this material right in this moment.

I am tempted to write a technical manual to accompany this book, with the purpose of sending it to every doctor who refuses to test and treat patients for *H pylori*. I have gathered so much scientific and medical research that I'm in danger of developing short-sightedness from reading so much! But I wanted to point out that it's not my intention to bombard you with detailed scientific explanations in this book because this would add further confusion to an already confusing topic.

It would be easy to get lost in the scientific information that is available on *H* pylori and confuse everyone! But in the end I hope the very basic science I present to help you understand just how important *H pylori* can be is balanced with my strong personal desire to help you. I hope the book fills the gaps that the medical system has left you with and that you are left in no doubt about the dangers of not dealing with *H pylori* even if when it is not causing obvious symptoms.

I want you to be able to use the diet and supplement programme immediately to regain optimal health, or at least a level of health that is acceptable and desirable for you. Finally, I want you to contact us with your story so that we can actively continue to push forward and spread this information far and wide with the end goal of helping everyone live healthier and happier lives.

If you'd like to send us your story please email it to office@hpexperts.com or post it on our forum at www.H-Pylori-Symptoms.com/forum

How To Use This Resource

Part One of this book has been written to help you understand the key issues around *H pylori* such as what it is, how it is transmitted from person-to-person, how to test for it and the symptoms it causes. I have laid out the information to answer the common questions that land in my Inbox on a daily basis in a way that will help you understand the problem at the appropriate level. To this end, I have only included the information that you *need* to know and have omitted complex technical detail.

I have included a great deal of information that your doctor will almost certainly not be aware of. Much of this information is critical if you are to make a full recovery from your infection and do not wish to pass the infection to your loved ones. It is not your doctor's fault if he or she does not understand *H pylori* in this amount of depth because doctors are there to help you with a wide range of health challenges rather than to specialise in one particular area. Research has indicated that doctors simply do not have time to read medical journals or research these specific topics in detail.

I feel that if you are to overcome *H pylori* successfully and keep it away, it is important that you understand why it is there in the first place, how it got there and why it is making you feel ill. Once you have this information, it makes it easier to overcome the problem.

Part Two of the book contains *The H Pylori Diet* and *Stomach Cleanse*. This programme contains a comprehensive list of foods that should be avoided in order to help you reduce inflammation in your digestive system, foods that commonly cause hidden allergies that can worsen your symptoms and foods that will help your system heal.

I also review the foods, herbs and supplements that are advertised on the Internet and in health food shops as being effective against *H pylori*. Needless to say, claims that some of these foods and herbs are miracle cures are highly exaggerated and so I teach you which ones work and which to avoid.

Finally, I teach you the supplement protocols that I have used successfully to help my clients overcome their *H pylori* – related symptoms. This section includes products that may inhibit *H pylori*, help you clear yeast and fungal overgrowth and replenish your digestive system with healthy bacteria. It also contains information on specific foods and products that can help your digestive lining heal.

It is important to understand that your symptoms may not clear immediately. If you have structural damage to your digestive system and resulting nutritional deficiencies, it may take some time for your symptoms to resolve. Think of it like this: if you go out in the sun all day without sunscreen, you may get badly burned. Just because you go inside, out of the sun, it doesn't mean that the sunburn is going to immediately disappear. Likewise, just because *H pylori* bacteria are not there anymore, it doesn't mean that the damage to your digestive lining will heal right away and as a result your symptoms may persist, sometimes for weeks or even months.

One of the most important aspects of the programme is to help you heal after you have cleared your infection. This is why I have included a comprehensive nutrition and lifestyle guide that teaches you the most common diet and lifestyle associated causes of symptoms so that you can work on these in order to strengthen your body against re-infection. I have seen *miraculous recoveries* in people who simply altered their diet to remove problem-causing foods.

Therefore, I highly recommend that you read through the entire book at least once before starting the programme. Take some time to absorb the information so that you are fully educated on the subject and what is required to ensure success. If you simply try to take a supplement that works against *H pylori*, you are missing the point and this may lead to re-infection or unsatisfactory results further down the line. The programme *will* work if you commit yourself to 90-days of good eating and taking the right supplements, at the right time and in the correct sequence.

Part One - Busting The *H Pylori* Myths

Introduction to Part One

During the course of the last three years, I've received a lot of emails and phone calls from people on the topic of *H pylori*. This is not unsurprising considering that I get more than one thousand people visiting the website each day and multiple thousands of online article and video views. I've also been fortunate to have worked with literally hundreds of people who have either had *H pylori*, or many of its symptoms. Because I had *H pylori* myself, I know a lot about *H pylori* from a 'patient's' perspective. I've also read a lot of research – many thousands of studies - from the scientific and medical community. From these 'human' and 'scientific' standpoints, I've reached several important conclusions:

- *H pylori* infection is a serious problem and it is hugely underestimated.

- Many doctors simply do not understand *H pylori*.

- Most of the excellent research that is being done around the world isn't reaching doctors who deal with patients.

- The Internet is rife with poor and incomplete information.

- The net result is that patients are confused and are not being heard, tested or treated properly in many cases.

The purpose of part one of *The H Pylori Diet* is to give an overview of *H pylori* and the problems it causes without entering into huge amounts of scientific detail. I want to empower you, not confuse you. My goal is to arm you with information that's actually going to be useful to you, such as how you acquire *H pylori*, the symptoms it causes and how to test for it, rather than the intricate biochemical workings of each individual 'genotype' of the bacteria!

What Is *Helicobacter Pylori*?

Helicobacter pylori, also known as H pylori, is a type of bacterium that lives primarily in your stomach and the upper part of your small intestine (the duodenum). *H pylori*, other species of *Helicobacter* bacteria and their DNA have also been isolated in the following parts of the body:

- Oral cavity / saliva / dental plaque
- Semen
- Vaginal tract
- Gallbladder
- Liver
- Colon
- Tonsils
- Salivary gland

H pylori bacteria have a corkscrew shape that enables them to bury into the lining of the stomach where they cause irritation, inflammation and damage to the delicate tissues of the upper digestive tract and possibly areas further down in the digestive 'tubing'.

H Pylori infection stimulates an immune response that can lead to degradation of the stomach lining tissue. Medical conditions that can result from this irritation and inflammation are gastritis, peptic and duodenal ulcers and even certain types of stomach cancer.

H Pylori can cause many digestive symptoms, including bloating, burping & belching, stomach pain, constipation, feeling of having a lump in the throat, acid reflux and constipation & diarrhoea. What your doctor probably won't tell you is that *H pylori* may also lead to chronic fatigue, sleep problems, back pain, skin diseases, headaches, nausea, weight gain and mood symptoms such as anxiety. It is now also heavily implicated in the development of insulin resistance, diabetes, high blood pressure and heart disease.

Figure 1: *Helicobacter pylori*

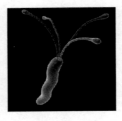

H pylori also has many 'brothers and sisters'. In fact, several *Helicobacter* species have been isolated in humans, including *H pullorum, H bilis, H hepaticus* and *H hartmann*i. It is not clear whether these species play a role in creating illness in humans although the scientific literature does suggest associations between some of these species and liver/gallbladder disease.

Similar bacteria have been found in animals, including cats, dogs, poultry, mice, pigs and even shellfish and dolphins. These findings have led some researchers to suggest that *H pylori* may be transmitted from animals to humans and possibly *vice versa*.

H pylori bacteria have been infecting humans for a very long time. Studies on 1,700 year-old Mummies in Chile's Atacama Desert revealed that our ancient relatives not only suffered from the same modern-day diarrhoeal parasites, such as *Cryptosporidium* and *Giardia*, but were also infected by *H pylori.*

Does Everyone Have *H pylori*?

Over the last three years I have received many emails from confused patients whose doctors have told them not to worry because "everyone has *H pylori*". However, thousands of medical studies and hundreds of stool test results from my clients' files prove that this is *simply not true*. It is not acceptable for patients to be diagnosed with *H pylori* only to be sent home under the premise that there's nothing wrong. As you'll see, *H pylori* infection can lead to a vast array of symptoms and is definitely involved in the development of some potentially serious medical conditions.

H pylori infection is widespread and is diagnosed worldwide. Its distribution is not uniform from location to location, however, and it is more prevalent in certain areas of the world than others. Depending on which book or study you read, it is estimated that *H pylori* infects between 50-70% of the world's population (3-5 billion people). There is a great deal of variation between infection rates in so-called 'developed' versus 'developing' countries. Table 1 provides an indication of infection rates in different geographical areas.

Continent	Country	Adult Infection Rate (%)
Africa	Algeria	43-92
	Kenya	94
	Nigeria	69-91
Asia / Australasia	China	86
	India	77-88
	Sri Lanka	72
	Thailand	74
	Australia	31
	New Zealand	7
Central America	Guatemala	58-65
	Mexico	60
Europe	Finland	34
	Italy	>40
	Spain	50-80
Middle East	Egypt	90
	Saudi Arabia	80
	Turkey	80-100
North America	USA	35-40
	Canada	20-40
South America	Argentina	38-62
	Brazil	82
	Chile	72
	Colombia	54-68

Table 1: Distribution of *H pylori* in Selected Countries (Adapted from Fleming, S. 2007, p.63)

What Causes H Pylori & Where Does It Come From?

As you can see from Table 1, the distribution of *H pylori* is closely related to a country's socioeconomic status. Higher rates of infection seem to be caused by:

- Birth in countries of lower socio-economic status

- Crowded living conditions

- Large families

- Unsanitary living conditions

- Unclean food or water

- Presence of babies/infants in the home

- Presence of pets in the home, especially cats and dogs

- Exposure to gastric contents of infected individuals (vomit)

- Late adult age group (45-65 years of age)

These risk factors provide us with clues as to how *H pylori* may be acquired or transmitted. Large families and overcrowding my predispose people to acquiring the infection from one another. Poor sanitary conditions may lead to exposure to food and water that has been contaminated by human or animal waste.

Is "Stress" A Risk Factor For Acquiring *H Pylori* Infection?

Most Functional Medicine doctors and practitioners would agree that if your body is under stress, or has been under stress recently, you are more likely to acquire a digestive infection such as *H pylori*. This is largely because mammals have a built-in stress response that ultimately leads to a reduction in the function of the digestive and immune systems, which in turn 'opens the door' for unwanted bacteria, parasites and fungal organisms to flourish.

When I ask my clients to complete their intake forms, I am always looking for a time-line of how their symptoms have developed. In many cases – too many to be coincidence - digestive problems develop during, or shortly after a period of stress. Common 'stressors' include:

- Money problems
- Divorce or relationship difficulties
- Redundancy
- Family bereavement
- Exams
- Car crash or other physical trauma
- Major infection
- Poor diet
- Chronic dehydration
- Too much or too little exercise
- Lack of sleep

With a depleted immune system, our bodies find it hard to fight infections, so the 'bugs' tend to become chronic and may remain in the digestive tract for many years – or even decades - before they're discovered. This is one reason why people (perhaps you!) suffer with chronic digestive symptoms, low energy, mood disorders and skin complaints for many years without ever understanding or discovering the cause.

Furthermore, as you will see later in this book, many people are astonished to find that, in addition to *H pylori*, they have other digestive infections, including bacteria such as *Salmonella, Clostridium difficile and E. coli*, fungal overgrowth with *Candida* and parasite infections such as *Blastocystis hominis, Giardia* and hookworm.

I have found that a person's diet is also a major cause of digestive symptoms. In fact, you may find that most, if not all of your symptoms, are caused by some of the common foods you are eating. Unfortunately most people are eating foods on a daily basis that are irritating the gut lining and creating exactly the same symptoms as infections like *H pylori*! These foods include gluten, soy and cow's milk.

This is the reason I designed the *H Pylori Diet* programme. Many customers have been amazed to find that even before they have taken treatment for *H pylori,* the simple act of altering their diet in accordance with the recommendations presented in this book completely resolves symptoms that they may have experienced for decades.

"I have lost about 30 lbs and feel better at age 66 than I did when I was in my 40's!!! The thing that I do not understand is that after all the years of digestive problems I was having, not once did any of the physicians ever mention this. At any rate, thanks again."

Tony Harras, California

Feel free to read and download our client intake forms at www.H-Pylori-Symptoms.com/consultation

Maggie, aged 75 and from South West England, explained to me that she had been experiencing digestive symptoms such as pain, bloating, wind and diarrhoea since she was a small child, seventy years ago. Recently, however, the symptoms had become much worse. Maggie was eventually diagnosed as having *H pylori* by her doctor shortly before Christmas 2009.

She was given FOUR consecutive courses of antibiotics, which I felt was a ridiculous regimen given her circumstances. The medications had not resolved any of her symptoms and had actually made her situation considerably *worse*, to the point where she had very severe diarrhoea and felt completely drained and exhausted, with very little appetite.

Digestive Symptoms

I've specialised in helping people overcome digestive complaints for more than three years now and in my experience the symptoms are most commonly caused by food intolerances and digestive infections. They are labeled "IBS" in the medical world, which can be a completely inaccurate and misleading diagnosis. Research clearly shows that reactions to foods like soy, sugar, cow's dairy and gluten can cause IBS and yet they are rarely mentioned in doctor's clinics. There is also overwhelming evidence that digestive infections also cause digestive symptoms.

Unfortunately, doctors do not tend to test for hidden infections unless patients are experiencing persistent vomiting or severe diarrhoea. Even when tests are performed, they are often lack the accuracy and sensitivity to miss the "bugs" and patients are told there is nothing there and that they will simply have to live with their symptoms for the rest of their lives. Maggie was no different.

Initial Test Results – 12th May, 2010

The findings of Maggie's test were very interesting and I knew right away that I was going be able to help her improve her health significantly. Maggie's results (below) indicated that her digestive system was home to FOUR different unwanted bugs: *H pylori*, *Blastocystis hominis*, *Endolimax nana* and a yeast/fungal overgrowth.

Pathogenic Bacteria	
Helicobacter pylori	7.0E+005 H
Clostridium difficile	<0.01
E.H.E. coli	<0.01
Campylobacter sp.	<0.01

Yeast/Fungi	
Yeast/Fungi; taxonomy unavailable.	+1 => 100 pg DNA/g specimen

A taxonomy unavailable finding may indicate ingested mold. The higher the number, the greater the indication for treatment, particularly when accompanied by clinical symptoms.

Parasites	
Blastocystis hominis	Positive
Endolimax nana	Positive

The fact that *H pylori* bacteria were still present was very interesting because Maggie had received four treatments with Triple Therapy antibiotics. Clearly the treatments had not worked. I was sure that the *H pylori* infection was still contributing to Maggie's symptoms, but I also knew that the other bugs we had found were also likely to be contributing to the problem.

Blastocystis hominis is a parasite that has been strongly associated with symptoms such as IBS (especially bloating and diarrhoea), depression, chronic fatigue and even arthritis.

It is a microscopic parasite that lives in the small intestine. I personally had *Blastocystis* as well as *H pylori* and so I have firsthand experience of the symptoms it can cause. *Endolimax nana* is another microscopic parasite: it is, in fact, an amoeba. Unfortunately it has not received much attention by researchers and is not generally recognised as a human pathogen.

Finally, Maggie's test result revealed that she had a light overgrowth of yeast and fungal organisms that had probably been caused by taking so many antibiotics for her *H pylori* infection. Maggie's +1 overgrowth indicated that she did not have severe overgrowth but this can often be misleading. If a person is very sensitive to toxins produced by yeast and fungal overgrowth, even a very light overgrowth or small imbalance can cause significant symptoms.

I always explain to my clients that it's actually a GOOD day when we find that they have digestive bugs because we finally know why they are not feeling well and exactly what we need to do in order to improve the situation.

I was convinced that the results went a long way to explaining why Maggie had been feeling unwell for such a long period of time. It was not clear exactly which "bug" was causing the most problems so I explained that it would be beneficial to work on cleansing all the unwanted invaders from Maggie's digestive system.

Phase One – First 30-Days

Maggie and I agreed that she would run a 30-day protocol, the same one, in fact, that is described in Part Two this book. I also recommended that Maggie stop consuming foods containing gluten and cow's milk. Remarkably, *her diarrhoea stopped as soon as she made these dietary adjustments*. It never ceases to amaze me how these simple dietary changes can bring such dramatic improvements and these are taught to you in Part Two of this book.

30-Days Later

We ran a follow-up consultation after the 30-day Stomach Cleanse protocol and Maggie reported that she was feeling much better. She mentioned that in addition to her dietary changes, she felt that taking Matula Herbal Formula had made a big difference. Despite her improvements, Maggie was still experiencing some discomfort. I advised that the likely reason for this would be the *Blastocystis* and *Endolimax* and we began a general parasite and yeast cleanse to deal with these issues.

Days 31-90

I've had great success in clearing the *Blastocystis* and *Endolimax* parasites using a specific herbal protocol that incorporates broad-spectrum anti-parasitic herbs in addition to the key diet changes. Specifically, I use *GI Microb-X and Oil of Oregano* from a wonderful company called *Designs For Health*. I do use other products from time to time, depending on the case, but these two products are my mainstays.

Our Next Consultation

Maggie emailed me enthusiastically to inform me that nearly all her symptoms had cleared. I suggested that we ought to run a consultation to discuss our next step. I was amazed that Maggie sounded like a completely new person when we spoke compared with the woman who first contacted me four months earlier! Her voice was loud and clear and she sounded fit, healthy and raring to go!

I recommended that we should definitely run a re-test using the GI Effects comprehensive stool test profile to make absolutely sure that the *H pylori, Blastocystis and Endolimax* had been eradicated.

Retest Results

Maggie's retest results revealed that the *H pylori*, yeast and fungal overgrowth and *Endolimax nana* were no longer present. The *Blastocystis* was still there, however, despite Maggie's symptoms improving dramatically. *Blastocystis* does not always cause symptoms. As with *H pylori*, there are different strains, some of which are believed to be problematic, with others being considered innocent 'passengers'.

You can see the retest result as well as several other real life case histories at **www.H-Pylori-Symptoms.com/case-histories**.

Summary & Learning Points

Maggie's case is a classic example of how extreme improvements in health can be accomplished, even when symptoms have been present for many years or even decades. It is a warming and inspiring story and I hope it encourages you to take action and break free from your symptoms.

It also highlights two areas that are of great concern for me. First, this lady had experienced symptoms for seventy years without ever being tested or correctly diagnosed. Second, she had been prescribed four courses of strong antibiotics in a very short space of time, despite the fact that her situation had been getting progressively worse after each course.

I lay no blame on anyone for these situations but it is my mission to educate and inspire you to break free from the belief that your doctor always has the knowledge required to resolve these situations. Unfortunately doctors do not necessarily receive specific training in parasitology and many do not realise that Triple Therapy antibiotics do not always eradicate *H pylori*.

How Does *H Pylori* Get Into Your Body?

The question "How did I become infected with *H pylori?"*
is one of the most popular emails that lands in our inbox.
Perhaps you are also confused about how *H Pylori* managed to
sneak into your stomach?

Here are two quotes from the very latest research emanating
from the *European Helicobacter Study Group's* 2010 literature
review:

> *All retrieved studies examining transmission of
> infection concluded that spread is from person to
> person.*

> *Currently the majority of available evidence points
> to the transmission of H pylori from human-to-
> human. The exact transmission from person-to-
> person is still unknown.*

These statements clearly indicate that scientists and
researchers agree on the fact that *H pylori* can be passed from
person-to-person. Why, then, do I receive so many emails from
confused people whose doctors have told them, *"don't be
silly... H pylori cannot be passed between people"*? Here is a
classic disconnect between doctor's knowledge and reality.

The consensus view within the literature is that *H pylori*
infections are acquired during childhood.

- A 2010 Turkish study reported a higher prevalence of
  H pylori in mothers with infected children compared to
  mothers with children who were not infected.

- A survey from the same year conducted in Brazil
  demonstrated that infected mothers were almost twenty
  times more likely to have an *H pylori* positive child.

- Finally a Greek study, also from 2010, reported that parents and siblings of children with *H pylori* were far more likely to be infected than in families of children who did not have the infection.

I can say without hesitation that my clinical experience supports the literature. I've found that *H pylori* can be present in spouses, sexual partners and children in the same household. I always recommend, therefore, that family members should be screened, especially when a client is finding it hard to eradicate *H pylori* using conventional treatment.

Wouldn't you agree that symptoms such as sickness, diarrhoea, abdominal pain and nausea are common in childhood and tend to be seen as 'the norm'? I can recall having a lot of heartburn, stomach cramps and constipation as a kid, but I didn't really complain about it because I thought it was 'normal'. In some people, these symptoms tend to disappear on their own, only to reappear and become chronic during adult years. I often wonder how many infections go undiagnosed in childhood and then cause potentially serious problems later on in life. Maggie's case history is a great case in point.

Unless childhood symptoms are severe, doctors tend not to test for infections. Instead, antibiotics or bed-rest are prescribed and as a result we do not discover which infection we actually have. Only when antibiotic treatments do not bring relief to symptoms do further investigations begin. It is certainly possible that *H pylori* could be the cause of many childhood symptoms that are considered to be part of the normal 'growing up' process.

H pylori, Kissing & Sexual Contact

Because H pylori and other *Helicobacter* species can inhabit the oral cavity (mouth) it is believed that they can be passed between people during kissing. The late Dr. William

Timmins, ND, suggested that up to 30% of *H pylori* infections could be passed through kissing. Although this has not been categorically proven, one study reported finding *H pylori* in the tonsil tissue of infected individuals and the authors concluded that their findings support the oral-oral transmission route.

In another study, it was found that spouses are often infected with exactly the same genetic strains of *H pylori*, again indicating that the infection is spread from person-to-person, *possibly* during intimate contact.

Dr. Timmins also isolated *H pylori* from semen. If *H pylori* can, indeed live in semen, it is possible that infection could occur during sexual intercourse or oral sex. *H pylori* bacteria and DNA have also been found in the vagina, alongside yeast species. Again, this indicates that perhaps sexual contact may play a role in transmission. Studies also indicate that *H pylori* may inhabit the large bowel, or colon, suggesting that anal sex could potentially lead to infection.

Sharing Eating & Drinking Utensils

Interestingly, it has been reported that *H pylori* bacteria have the ability to survive on chopsticks, indicating that the sharing of eating and drinking utensils, water bottles, toothbrushes and other oral implements may also be a transmission route. Researchers found that even when chopsticks were washed, *H Pylori* could still be isolated from them.

Mother to Child & Family Transmission

As indicated previously, scientists believe that the mother to child transmission route is a likely cause of infection. It has been shown that *H pylori* strains in infant infections often match the exact genetic strains carried by the Mother. One study concluded that:

"The detection of H pylori in mother's dental plaque seems to be a critical factor for the intrafamilial spread."

The authors of a 2005 study found that the likelihood of a child acquiring an infection was much higher if the mother was infected versus the father.

Finally, a study conducted among Amazonian natives in Brazil showed that the *H pylori* acquisition rate was 25% in early childhood. In other words, the infection rate in very young children was approximately one quarter. In this study 50% of children aged 2 were infected, at 15 years 86.1% were infected and almost 100% of the adults had *H pylori*.

Despite the likelihood of the mother-infant route being an important transmission route, I have not yet found any evidence that supports breastfeeding as a mode of transmission, though some experts have commented that the wetting of the mother's nipple with her saliva prior to breast feeding may lead to infection of the infant.

H Pylori in Water

Studies indicate that *H pylori* can survive in water and that drinking contaminated water is a source of *H pylori* infection in humans. For example, *H pylori* bacteria have been found in well water, seawater that is close to sewerage outlets and on vegetables that have been treated with water contaminated with faecal matter.

As I mentioned in my introduction, I believe I acquired my *H pylori* infection in 2004 whilst on holiday in Egypt. I had terrible heartburn, nausea and vomiting for two days and then diarrhoea symptoms for around a week. After the first week I developed a *Candida* overgrowth that covered my tongue white/yellow and suffered with fatigue and short spells of nausea for many weeks. Whilst I am unable to pinpoint the exact route of transmission it appears likely that I consumed contaminated water, ice or food.

H Pylori in Food

Studies have demonstrated that lettuce washed in water contaminated with faeces may contain *H pylori*. *H pylori* may also be acquired by eating poorly cooked foods, especially meat, poultry and eggs. A recent report by the British Government asserted that eggs from caged hens contain a higher level of *Salmonella* bacteria compared to eggs from organically raised hens. It is certainly reasonable to suspect that poorer quality eggs and other foods may contain higher levels of *H pylori*. Dr. Michael Liebowitz DC believes that poor quality eggs are a source of *H pylori* infection.

It has been shown that *H pylori* can be picked up by houseflies and it is reasonable to assume that flies that have been in contact with human or animal waste may pose a threat of infection. Food contaminated with cockroach excretions has also been identified as another possible mode of transmission.

Hospitals & Endoscopic Procedures

An endoscopy procedure involves the passing of a tube down the throat of the patient. The tube has a camera on the end that allows the doctors to see structural damage in the stomach such as stomach inflammation (gastritis), ulcers, tumours and hernias. Medical opinion, as well as some research has shown that *H pylori* can be spread using contaminated equipment. This is somewhat ironic – a testing method for *H Pylori* can actually *cause* the infection!

Pets & Other Animals

Many species of *Helicobacter* have been identified and in a wide variety of animals, including cats, dogs, sheep, gerbils, rabbits, monkeys, cows, pigs, tigers, cheetahs, poultry, wild birds and even dolphins and sharks. Some scientists believe that certain *Helicobacter* species may be passed from animals to humans, a process known as *zoonosis*.

To my knowledge, this hypothesis has not yet been fully confirmed, though it is likely that some transmission does occur.

Yeast Organisms

Helicobacter species can survive in yeast colonies that inhabit the mouths of dogs and cats. It is plausible, therefore, that allowing pets to lick our hands and face, or even petting areas of the animal that have been licked, may lead to the transmission of the *Helicobacter* organisms from the animals to humans.

There is a definite relationship between yeast organisms and *H pylori*. Some scientists believe that yeasts actually harbour *H pylori*. It is also proven that *H pylori* and yeast overgrowth – often known as *Candida albicans* - can occur at the same time. *Candida* can actually cause the same or very similar symptoms as *H Pylori*.

When Triple Therapy antibiotics are used against *H pylori*, stomach levels of *Candida albicans* have been shown increase by around 30%. This is one of the major disadvantages of using antibiotics against *H Pylori*.

Research also demonstrates that when proton pump inhibitors and other antacid drugs are used to reduce stomach acid, reflux and heartburn, *Candida* organisms also spread rapidly. This has enormous implications because *Candida* overgrowth can also cause or contribute to a vast array of symptoms and health problems. 'Rebound' overgrowth of *Candida* as well as other yeast and fungal organisms is an extremely common reason why symptoms do not improve, or even worsen following treatment for *H pylori*.

Many times I have found that a client's symptoms have been a combination of *H pylori* and *Candida*. On other occasions, I have found that yeast and fungal overgrowth alone was causing the symptoms - digestive discomfort, constipation, diarrhoea, heartburn, painful gums or tongue, headaches and other common symptoms.

Summary

In summary, although no *precise* mechanism has been established to explain how *H pylori* infection is acquired, there appear to be several important modes of transmission:

- Person-to-person – possibly through kissing, sharing eating and drinking utensils and sexual contact.

- Being in contact with the vomit or stools of an infected person, for example in day care centres & hospitals.

- Drinking water that has been contaminated with faeces.

- Eating food that has been contaminated by tainted water or flies and cockroaches.

- Zoonosis (animal to human).

- In hospitals via infected diagnostic equipment.

Can You Pass *H Pylori* To Your Children & Loved Ones?

Most doctors will tell you that *H pylori* is not contagious. However I believe this to be completely false. As you've seen, studies show that spouses are often infected by the same strain of *H pylori* and that a mother can pass *H pylori* to her children.

Whilst it is not guaranteed that you will not pass *H pylori* to other people, I want you to be aware that the possibility of doing so exists.

Joyce had been suffering with chronic digestive symptoms for some twenty years. When we ran a stool antigen test, we found that she had an active *H pylori* infection. I recommended that Paul, her husband, should also be tested. If Joyce worked hard to clear her infection, but Paul was also carrying the infection, he may pass it right back to her. Paul's results also came back positive. I put both Joyce and Paul on a two-month course of antimicrobial herbs and also recommended some dietary adjustments to help reduce digestive inflammation. We then waited four weeks to retest. To their relief, both Joyce and Paul tested negative for *H pylori* and their symptoms had largely improved. Joyce actually found complete remission from her symptoms only after she had also altered her diet to eliminate key foods that were creating IBS. We then ran a test for their daughter, Jenny. Guess what? She also had *H pylori!*

I always recommend that *all family members* run testing if one member is diagnosed with *any* digestive invader. This may be difficult to justify because *H pylori* and other digestive infections do not always cause symptoms. But when one family member works hard to eradicate their infection and the others are not tested, it might be unwittingly passed right back to them resulting in confusion, wasted time, energy and sometimes money.

What Are The Symptoms of *H Pylori*?

- Do you have bloating, belching or burping?
- Do you suffer with acid reflux?
- Does your stomach hurt or burn?
- Do you get chest or upper back pain?
- Are you constipated?
- Do you feel tired all the time?
- Is it hard to fall or stay asleep?

- Do you sometimes feel like you have an uncomfortable lump in your throat?
- Has your doctor told you that you have IBS?
- Do you get headaches?
- Are you losing or gaining weight for no reason?
- Do you have rosacea, hives or urticaria?
- Do you experience nausea, especially in the mornings?

These are just *some* of the symptoms that I have seen improve dramatically or even disappear when people change their diet and eradicate *H pylori*. Unfortunately, the link between foods, hidden digestive infections and bacterial imbalances and these symptoms are not always recognised.

Some of the symptoms of *H pylori* are obvious – reflux, stomach pain, belching and burping - and will tend to be acknowledged by medical staff, but others are subtle and may seem to be completely unrelated to the digestive system. But make no mistake, *H Pylori* has the potential to cause or contribute to unwanted symptoms in many parts of your body and it is heavily implicated in the development of 'dis-ease'.

Laura, 49, had fatigue and female hormone symptoms such as depression, anxiety and painful periods (PMS). She also had some digestive issues, including bloating and diarrhoea. Her symptoms had been present for many years. Laura had never been tested for digestive bugs so we ran a stool antigen test, which revealed that she had *H pylori*. I recommended that Laura follow anti-inflammatory diet and she immediately felt better, with lots more energy. I then recommended that she take a 30-day course of Matula Herbal Formula. Within 60-days of beginning the programme, approximately half of Laura's symptoms had cleared. We then re-tested, using a different stool test. The *H pylori* had gone, but the test showed that she had a parasite, and a tricky one at that. Laura had *whipworm*. We ran a very strong course of anti-parasitic herbs for 60-days, and Laura emailed me to say that her 'deep' energy levels, as she described them, had returned and her digestion was completely back to normal.

One of the most confusing things about *H pylori* is that it does not cause obvious symptoms in everyone. In fact, some carriers of *H pylori* are completely asymptomatic, meaning that they have no symptoms at all. Others may have mild, long-term symptoms such as stomach pain, bloating, skin rashes and general low energy. Others still may be rushed to the emergency room with severe chest pains, nausea, vomiting and diarrhoea. To make matters even more complicated, in some people, *H pylori* infection does not cause *any* of the common digestive symptoms but *can* lead to symptoms such as depression and anxiety.

Whether people experience symptoms from *H pylori* seems to depend on several factors:

- The severity of the infection – how many *H pylori* organisms are present?

- The particular strain of *H pylori* causing the infection – there are many different strains.

- The length of time the infection has been present.

- 'Host' factors, including genetic susceptibility, smoking, stress levels, food sensitivity and nutritional status.

H pylori infection creates a very complex set of interactions with the infected person's gut lining and immune system. It's too complicated to go into detail here and, frankly, the level of depth in some of the molecular biology is too complex even for me to comprehend! But whether you experience symptoms as a result of having any infection is largely the result of your body's interaction with that particular bug. Because we have so much genetic variability as humans and because there are so many strains of *H pylori*, you simply need to understand that the infection will not affect everyone in the same way.

Digestive Symptoms Caused By *H Pylori*

The most obvious symptoms of *H pylori* infection occur in the digestive system and the bacteria are known to cause the following symptoms:

- Heartburn (burning sensation in throat and stomach areas)

- Acid Reflux

- Chest pain and pain between the shoulder blades

- Belching and burping

- Excessive gas

- Abdominal bloating and cramps

- Constipation

- Diarrhoea

- Gastritis (inflammation of the stomach)

Acute Symptoms

Some people develop severe, *acute* symptoms. These are usually characterised by nausea, vomiting, severe chest pains, heartburn, extreme fatigue and diarrhoea. It is not uncommon for people to report feeling like they are having a 'heart attack' when a severe acute infection is acquired and this is not dissimilar to the way I felt in 2004, when I believe I acquired my *H pylori* infection in Egypt.

Chronic Symptoms

H pylori infections can also cause *chronic* symptoms. These are usually less severe and tend towards mild digestive discomfort such as bloating, indigestion, constipation and mild heartburn or reflux. Infected individuals may also feel tired, low in mood, have headaches and generally 'not feel themselves'. These are some of the most difficult symptoms to figure out because doctors are not inclined to consider digestive infections as a cause of non-digestive symptoms.

Is *H Pylori* The Same As Irritable Bowel Syndrome (IBS)?

This is a question I'm often asked and it opens up a can of worms! Irritable bowel syndrome is a big topic to cover and is deserving of an entire book. What I will say at this stage is that any chronic, hidden digestive infection – including *H* pylori - can cause the symptoms often labelled as IBS.

IBS stands for "Irritable Bowel Syndrome" and it's a blanket term for a whole bunch of digestive complaints. In my opinion, it's a 'get out clause' diagnosis that is used to fob patients off when symptoms are present but their cause is unknown. Whilst there are some true cases of IBS out there, where biochemical imbalances within the body are causing problems with neurological control of the intestines, most cases of so-called IBS can be explained by two things:

1. **Food** – if you have digestive symptoms, common foods will almost certainly be contributing to you not feeling well. This issue is covered in the second half of the book. I have designed *The H Pylori Diet* to help you avoid all the common foods that can cause the same symptoms as IBS and *H Pylori*.

2. **Infections** – *H pylori* is one of many digestive infections that can cause IBS-like symptoms. Others include parasites, opportunistic bacteria such as *Salmonella, Vibrio, Aeromonas* and *Pseudomonas*, pathogenic bacteria such as *E. coli* and *Campylobacter* or yeast and fungal overgrowth.

If you have been diagnosed with 'IBS' and your doctor has told you there is no cure, I urge you to have faith. Your symptoms will almost certainly improve if you follow *The H Pylori Diet* and run a comprehensive stool panel to identify which infections you have and how well you are digesting your food.

Fatigue, Mood, Sleep & Weight Management Problems

H pylori may cause, or at least contribute to, many symptoms outside the digestive system. These symptoms are known as 'extragastric manifestations' of *H pylori*. Research is uncovering associations with more and more extragastric symptoms and diseases. Some of the most common symptoms include:

- Depression & anxiety
- Low energy
- Lethargy
- Heart palpitations
- Brain fog
- Headaches
- Sleep problems
- Rapid weight loss

- Weight gain
- Skin problems such as urticaria and rosacea
- Bad breath
- Pain between the shoulder blades
- Sinus problems

When we take the time to understand how our bodies work, it is easy to see how *H pylori* infection may lead to symptoms outside our digestive system. Science is now uncovering some very interesting links between *H pylori* and seemingly unrelated symptoms and health conditions. Whilst an 'association' does not mean that *H pylori* infection *causes* these symptoms and diseases, it suggests that the infection may play a role in their development, or aetiology:

- Anaemia
- Bronchitis
- Colitis
- Colorectal Cancer
- Crohn's Disease
- Halitosis
- Heart Disease
- High Blood Pressure
- High Cholesterol / Lipid Imbalances
- Homocysteine
- Hypochloridia (low stomach acid)
- Gallstones
- Insulin Resistance
- Liver Disease
- Lung Cancer
- Migraines
- Osteoporosis
- Pancreatitis
- Parkinson's Disease
- Raynaud's Syndrome
- Rosacea
- Sperm Health / Male Fertility
- Thyroid (autoimmune)
- Type I Diabetes
- Urticaria
- Vitamin and Mineral Deficiency
- Vomiting during Pregnancy
- Weight gain / obesity

Cris, from London, came to me complaining of male hormonal problems, including loss of libido. He had very mild bloating symptoms and no obvious signs of a digestive infection. We ran stool antigen testing and discovered that he had *H pylori*. We also ran a urine test to check for nutrient deficiencies and liver function, which showed a deficiency in amino acids (protein building blocks). These nutritional deficiencies are common because *H pylori* can lead to a reduction stomach acid production. With low stomach acid, it is hard to digest and absorb these nutrients properly. Amino acids are important building blocks for many chemicals, including those that influence mood and libido. I recommended a natural protocol to help with the *H pylori* (confirmed negative on retest) along with an anti-inflammatory diet. Cris also took some supplements to replenish the missing nutrients and within 6-months had made excellent progress.

Whilst this list is not exhaustive, it illustrates the weird and wonderful effects that a simple digestive infection can have on other areas of the body. It also shows you how much research is being conducted in the area, most of which the majority of doctor's know nothing about. Let's take a more detailed look at some specific 'extragastric' conditions that are now being associated with *H pylori* infection.

H pylori & Skin Disease

I've been arguing for years that digestive infections cause and contribute significantly to skin problems. We know that dandruff, jock itch and athlete's foot are fungal problems and that dermatitis herpitiformis is caused by gluten, a sticky protein in some grains that has its own section later in *The H Pylori Diet*. I have observed a vast array of rashes, blemishes, sores and other skin problems simply go away when we have worked on clients' digestive health.

Around Christmas 2009, I read a fantastic review paper in the *European Journal of Dermatology* that pulled together a great deal of research linking *H pylori* with skin diseases. It added scientific validation to all my observations.

The paper suggests a link between *H pylori* and various skin conditions, including:

- Rosacea
- Urticaria / Hives
- Atopic Dermatitis
- Psoriasis
- Immune Thrombocytopenic Purpura (ITP)
- Sjogren's Syndrome
- Pruritis
- Prurigo

Of all these skin diseases, the strongest associations are between *H pylori*, urticaria, rosacea and ITP. I have personally observed rapid improvements in rosacea in clients when they successfully eradicated *H pylori*, improvements in dermatitis when they stopped eating gluten and improvements in psoriasis when they eradicated parasites and fungal overgrowth.

If you'd like further information on *H pylori* and its relationship with skin disease I highly recommend that you visit **www.H-Pylori-Symptoms.com/skin-diseases**.

Can *H Pylori* Cause Heart Disease?

Scientists are uncovering evidence that certain infections – including *H pylori* – may contribute to heart disease and strokes. Other infections such as *Cytomegalovirus* and *Chlamydia pneumoniea* are also implicated. Several complex mechanisms have been proposed to help explain how *H pylori* infection leads to the development of these serious conditions. I'll keep the explanations brief and simple for you but please do not underestimate the importance of this section.

I've read more than thirty studies where associations between *H pylori* and heart disease were noted. It's important to understand that an association does not represent a direct cause and effect relationship. What the data tell us are that in general:

- Certain strains of *H pylori* - especially one called 'Cag-A' - are found in more people who have certain types of heart disease than in those who do not.

- Coronary heart disease may be more severe in people who are infected with *H pylori*

- *H pylori* infection seems to increase the rate of atherosclerosis, or the build-up of plaque in the arteries.

- Susceptibility to ischemic strokes seems to be related to *H pylori* infection.

- Certain strains of *H pylori* – Cag-A again - seem to increase the risk of patients suffering a heart attack or stroke.

- Eradication of *H pylori* leads to improvement of plaque levels in arterial walls.

- *H pylori* may be related to the incidence of atrial fibrillation (heart palpitations).

I think you probably get the picture. However, I have more for you! As you may be aware, a number of other diseases and 'advanced' clinical conditions are closely related to heart disease. These include high cholesterol and imbalanced lipid profiles, high blood pressure and insulin resistance, all of which seem to be strongly related to one major factor: inflammation.

I'd like to discuss inflammation on its own in a little more detail because, as most experts who are worth listening to agree, inflammation is the new *"Mother of Disease"*.

H pylori infection always causes inflammation. It doesn't matter whether you can feel the inflammation or not, it's *always* there if you have *H pylori*. If you look at the literature, you'll see quotes such as:

> *Virtually all H pylori positive subjects develop chronic active gastritis.*

> *As first reported by Robin Warren, the presence of Helicobacter pylori is always associated with an inflammation of the underlying gastric mucosa as evidenced by an infiltration of inflammatory cells.*

Gastritis is inflammation of the stomach and duodenitis is inflammation of the small intestine. *H pylori* can live in the stomach for months, years and even decades without causing any symptoms whatsoever. It can, of course, just as easily cause symptoms that give it away, such as stomach pain, heartburn, acid reflux, belching, bloating, nausea and vomiting. But the point I'd like to make is that even when symptoms are not present, it seems as though *H pylori* can cause hidden damage which may lead to significant pathology elsewhere in the body. This is the area of most concern for me because doctors will generally not test and treat patients unless the common *H pylori* symptoms are present.

When inflammation is present in the body, serum levels of a chemical called C-reactive protein (CRP) tend to elevate. CRP is an acute phase protein that is made by the body as a kind of protective mechanism in response to inflammation, independent of where in the body the inflammation is. CRP is also strongly correlated with the development of heart disease and, in fact, is used as a marker for cardiovascular risk assessment.

Let's look at the relationship of *H pylori* infection to CRP:

- Serum CRP levels appear to be higher in subjects with *H pylori*.

- CRP levels seem to decrease in studies where *H pylori* is eradicated.

So it does appear that CRP levels increase in *H pylori* infection and, because CRP is independently associated with the future risk of coronary heart disease and stroke, the inflammatory response created by *H pylori* appears to be a factor in the development of those diseases.

Recent research has also provided information linking *H pylori* to high blood pressure and insulin resistance. Insulin resistance is a pre-cursor to type II diabetes, which itself is strongly associated with inflammation. Here are some of the research findings that 'thicken the plot':

- *H pylori* seems to have an effect on the daily blood glucose fluctuation in patients with type II diabetes.

- *H pylori* infection appears to be a risk factor for insulin resistance.

- In some studies, infection with *H pylori* seems to independently cause insulin resistance.

- The eradication of *H pylori* appears to help lower blood pressure.

- *H pylori* infection is significantly associated with the metabolic syndrome, a 'syndrome' which leads to insulin resistance and heart disease.

- *H pylori* infection is associated with elevated serum cholesterol levels.

- The eradication of *H pylori* can help to normalize serum lipid profiles (this is the relationship between HDL and LDL cholesterol).

I realise that this is beginning to get a little complicated now and I don't want to confuse you. Suffice to say that the metabolic changes that may accompany *H pylori* can lead to complications that, for some people, may become serious.

Another reason I wanted to share this information about inflammation relates to the seemingly unrelated every day symptoms that so many people complain of. In a study published in 2008, researchers induced inflammation in several groups of patients by administering a natural pro-inflammatory chemical, interferon-gamma. Again, without going into enormous amounts of scientific detail, patients developed the following symptoms:

**If you would like to access a full scientific
and medical reference list please visit
www.H-Pylori-Symptoms.com/h-pylori-studies**

Table 1. Overlapping of symptoms of acute sickness behaviour associated with IFN-α therapy and the somatic symptoms in MDD

Symptoms	Prevalence in IFN-α therapy [a], %	Prevalence in MDD[b], %
Fatigue/asthenia	39–90	73
Headache	27–67	33[e]
Gastrointestinal symptoms	50[c, 1]	34–47[f]
Psychomotor slowing	40[c]	59–65[f]
Insomnia	20–39[d]	63
Irritability	35[d]	50
Arthralgia	9–36	31[e]
Musculoskeletal pain	26–32	62–80[g, 2]
Abdominal pain	15–20	21[e]
Anorexia	13–19	40
Anxiety	13–18[d]	57
Poor concentration	14[d]	51

Table Copied from Su, K-P. Neurosig. 2009;17:144-152.

It's my hope that you realise how important inflammation is in creating every day symptoms. Take a look at the table above and note whether you experience any of these symptoms. I'm sure some of them are a little too familiar for comfort! I'd like to point out that I am certainly not blaming every symptom on inflammation caused by *H pylori*. *Any* symptom can have different causes in different people. But wouldn't you agree that the evidence to support the role of *H pylori* in so many symptoms and metabolic diseases is compelling? Also consider that we're only talking about one of many hidden chronic digestive infections that do not get the medical attention they deserve.

My personal experience of having *H pylori* along with my clinical observations support the notion that *H pylori* infection is at least involved in many of the common symptoms listed above. But it is actually the *response* of the human body to the infection that creates the symptoms we experience, in the same way as it's our immune system's response to a common cold that causes the blocked nose, coughing, elevated temperature and swollen glands we've all experienced!

My advice to you is to look at your health history and symptoms:

- Do you experience, or have you experienced symptoms that haven't been explained properly?

- Have you actually run any tests to determine reasons why you have those symptoms?

- Even if you have had a negative *H pylori* test, perhaps you are reacting to common foods that you're eating, or perhaps you have other digestive infections?

Fortunately, the *H Pylori Diet* has been specifically designed to give you a basic nutrition plan that has anti-inflammatory qualities. In fact, the whole purpose of the programme is to help reduce inflammation in your digestive tract so that your treatments for *H pylori* become more effective. I also invite you to contact our offices to enquire about our advanced online *Health Freedom Secrets* programme, lab testing and phone consultancy services. Just email **Office@HPExperts.com**.

H Pylori & Stomach Ulcers

The spotlight fell on *H pylori* in 2005, when two doctors were awarded the Nobel Prize for Physiology and Medicine for finally proving that *H pylori causes* stomach, or 'peptic', ulcers. The award was the culmination of some twenty years' work on the part of Dr. Barry Marshall, who first proposed a link between *H pylori* and ulcers in the mid nineteen-eighties.

Peptic ulcer disease is a well-known complication of chronic *H pylori* infection. It is estimated that approximately 15-20% of *H pylori* carriers develop ulcers. Whilst this may seem like a small percentage, remember that at least half the world's population carries *H pylori* and that 20% of that 3 billion equals 600,000,000 people!

It's also estimated that around 80% stomach ulcers and >90% duodenal ulcers are caused by *H pylori*. Other causes and risk factors involved in the development of ulcers include the use of aspirin and other NSAID medications, tobacco smoking, alcohol consumption, stress and diet. Therefore, *H pylori* eradication will not always bring about ulcer healing.

The most common complication of peptic ulcer disease is bleeding. According to De Vries and Kuipers, approximately 10-20% of people who have *H pylori* related ulcers develop a bleeding, or perforated ulcer. A bleeding ulcer is a serious medical condition that requires immediate attention.

Bleeding Ulcer Checklist:

- Dark, tarry stools
- Vomit with 'coffee-like granules'
- Vomit with blood
- Gnawing pain between breastbone and naval
- Severe nausea
- Weakness
- Anaemia and low red cell count on blood test
- Occult blood in stool analysis

I recommend that you seek medical assistance immediately if you experience these symptoms, especially those involving dark, tarry stools, blood or granules in vomit or severe nausea and burning sensations.

H Pylori Can Cause Stomach Cancer

I am dumbfounded when I hear tales of doctors telling patients *"everyone has H pylori, it's not a problem"*. We've already seen that *H pylori* infection likely contributes to certain metabolic imbalances that lead to insulin resistance, high blood pressure, the metabolic syndrome and heart disease and that it certainly causes stomach inflammation and ulcers that can perforate and cause major problems. We also know that *H pylori* infection also plays a role in certain types of stomach cancer.

In the 1990s, the *World Health Organisation* classified *H pylori* as a *Class I Carcinogen*. This classification puts *H pylori* at the same level of risk for stomach cancer as cigarette smoking is for lung cancer. Two excerpts from the European Study Group's review of gastric carcinogenesis emphasise the importance of *H pylori* and lifestyle factors in the development of gastric cancers:

> *Several environmental factors, including Helicobacter pylori infection, consumption of salted and nitrated foods, and cigarette smoking, have been found to be associated with the risk of developing gastric cancer.*

> *Although the incidence of gastric cancer differs between continents, the infection with Helicobacter pylori is the most important risk factor in all geographic areas and H pylori infection carries the same risk for both histologic types of gastric cancer and diffuse type. Several studies in the last year have gained further evidence that eradication of the bacteria is one of the most promising preventative strategies in the fight against gastric cancer.*

Whilst these statements sound scary, gastric cancer is thought to develop in only around 1-3% of *H pylori*-infected individuals. Still, this means that for every one million people with an *H pylori* infection, ten thousand will develop gastric cancer. Is it really worth the risk?

As I am not a cancer expert, it is not my place to enter into a detailed discussion on the topic. But if your doctor is not listening to you, or is fobbing you off with the notion that *H* pylori is harmless, please take this book to him or her and refer to the scientific validation from the 2010 literature at **www.Helicobacter.org.**

The final point I'd like to make about this topic is that the earlier *H pylori* is dealt with, the better:

> *H pylori eradication prevents gastric cancer development and it seems the earlier the bacteria get eradicated, the more significant the decrease of gastric cancer risk.*

If we can reduce the risk and incidence of gastric cancer by eradicating *H pylori*, do you think it's likely that we can also reduce the risk of all the other symptoms and illnesses discussed so far? The problem is that our medical model waits until the symptoms and diseases have already developed before intervening. We are told to ignore and 'live with' the minor symptoms we experience until one day they develop into severe symptoms like ulcers, diabetes and as we've seen, cancer and heart disease!

In Part Two of this book, *The H Pylori Diet* gives you the tools to help you overcome *H pylori* and in doing so, there's a good chance that you may reduce your cancer risk. As well as teaching you how you can safely eradicate *H pylori*, the programme also teaches you how to adapt your diet and lifestyle to reduce inflammation and speed up the healing of your entire digestive system.

Can *H Pylori* Kill?

As you've seen, we really need a reality check with *H pylori*. Infection can cause serious complications that may lead to death. However we must acknowledge that these complications may not be solely caused by *H pylori* alone. Gastric cancers have causes other than *H pylori* and it is believed that only a very small percentage of *H* pylori infected people will develop cancer as a result of the infection.

Insulin resistance, heart disease and other metabolic complications of inflammation are not the sole result of *H pylori* infection either. Diet, nutritional status, lifestyle, stress, other infections and many other factors determine the development and outcomes of these diseases. However, as we've seen, the presence of *H pylori* definitely contributes to these and other more serious conditions, so it must never be underestimated.

If you have *H pylori,* you can avoid all these complications by simply making sure that you receive effective therapy. If you are experiencing symptoms, the causes of which have not been identified, then seek testing by speaking with your doctor, or use the resources presented in this book. My team of practitioners can quickly help you identify the cause(s) of your symptoms and help you move back towards optimal health. This brings us nicely onto the next section.

What Tests Are Available For *H Pylori*?

I receive dozens of emails each week asking me about *H pylori* testing. Here is a list of the most common problems people face when it comes to getting tested for *H pylori*. Perhaps you have experienced some of these difficulties?

- There is great inconsistency in doctors' willingness to test.

- There is a degree of inconsistency in the accuracy of testing.

- It can be very hard to get a second test if you feel that the first one was inaccurately reported.

- Certain types of testing may not be accessible in your area.

- Doctors may not be aware that certain types of testing even exist. For example some doctors do not know about stool testing for *H pylori*.

- Budgetary or insurance restrictions, depending on the country you're in, may hamper attempts to access tests.

- You may have to wait weeks or even months to be tested.

- Retests are performed too soon after completing antibiotic therapy and the wrong type of test is used to confirm eradication.

I've come across all these problems in my work and it can be incredibly frustrating. However in my opinion, there is an even bigger limitation to conventional *H pylori* testing, which is that the procedures *only* test for *H pylori*. I'd like to draw to your attention something of great importance: *H pylori* has many cousins, most of which are capable of causing the same, similar or even worse symptoms than *H pylori* itself. Other bacteria, parasites and yeast overgrowth can all be confused with *H pylori* symptoms. Yet the medical system sees it fit to ignore these other infections for the most part even while they are wreaking havoc on your body!

There are four main tests for *H pylori*. The relative advantages and disadvantages of these tests are listed in the table below.

A Summary of the Advantages and Disadvantages of Testing Methods for *H pylori*

TEST	ADVANTAGES	DISADVANTAGES
Blood Antibody Test A blood sample is taken and analysed for antibodies to *H pylori*. This test is looking for your body's reaction to the infection, not the *H pylori* organism *per se*	• Can be helpful in identifying H pylori initially.	• May lead to false positive results because antibodies can be present even when infection is gone. • Should not be used to retest after treatment. • Involves blood draw and may be stressful to patient. • Requires visit to clinic.
Urea Breath Test (UBT) Patients blow into a bag and the air is analysed for gases that are produced when *H pylori* is living in the gut.	• Relatively easy to perform • Non-invasive • High accuracy is reported in the medical literature.	• May miss low-level infections, such as those in children. • May miss infection following antibiotic treatment if test is performed too soon. • Experientially, positive results may be reported when *H pylori* not present, but fungal overgrowth is.

Test	Advantages	Disadvantages
Endoscopy / Biopsy A tube is inserted into the mouth and passed down the throat into the stomach. A camera is used to identify inflammation, ulcers and hernias. A biopsy may be taken of the stomach tissue and analysed for *H pylori*.	• Can identify ulcers & gastritis. • Can identify hernias, which may cause reflux and burning symptoms.	• Invasive, stressful & uncomfortable. • Requires visit to clinic. • Can actually lead to *H pylori* infection (research has shown that *H pylori* can survive on the equipment and be passed from person to person).
Stool Antigen Test One or more stool samples are taken and analysed for H pylori antigens (fragments of the cell wall of the bacteria)	• High accuracy. • Can identify many other infectious agents (parasites, bacteria, yeast) • Convenient & can be done at home. • Excellent for retesting.	• Some tests may miss the organisms if multiple samples are not taken. • Samples may degrade during transportation. • Variation in quality of laboratories.

What Is The Best Test For *H Pylori*?

This is as very difficult question to answer because there is no 'right or wrong'. Each test has merits and drawbacks. The most important point I'd like you to take from this section is that a negative test result from *any* of these tests does not necessarily mean that *H pylori* is not present. All the tests can provide false-negatives. It is also known that the blood and breath tests can also provide false positives, where *H pylori* is reported as being present when, in fact, it is not.

Graeme contacted my office informing me that his 9 year old son, Brodie, had suffered with 2 months of symptoms, starting with nausea, vomiting, constipation, reflux, motion sickness and weight loss. He was unable to concentrate at school and was indeed having to take time off. He had taken a blood test and breath test for *H pylori*, both of which had come back negative. When we ran a stool test, we found *H pylori* and Brodie was able to overcome his symptoms quickly.

In my practice I run comprehensive stool testing with my clients. Whilst there is an ongoing debate about which *H pylori* test is the most accurate, stool testing carries one major benefit: you can assess the stool sample for a multitude of markers in a single test. The level of information you can ascertain from a single stool test is infinitely more helpful than a single marker for *H pylori* and the testing can be done in the comfort of your own home.

The advantages of running comprehensive stool testing are as follows:

✓ From a single stool sample you can identify more than thirty different bacteria, parasites and fungal organisms that may be causing problems.

✓ Examples of these organisms include *Salmonella, Clostridium difficile, Camylobacter, E. coli, Giardia,*

Blastocystis hominis, amoebas, hookworm, whipworm, pinworm, *Candida albicans* and many more.

✓ You can identify whether your friendly or 'predominant' bacteria are present in optimal balance (these friendly 'bugs' are often referred to as *probiotics*).

✓ You're able to check for gluten-intolerance, inflammation and immune function within your intestines.

✓ You can check to see whether you are producing enough digestive enzymes and whether you're digesting and absorbing dietary fat, protein and carbohydrate.

In many cases, I've helped clients identify why they've been plagued by symptoms, sometimes for decades, simply by having them run the comprehensive stool analysis. It's very important to remember that *H pylori* is not the only unwanted visitor lurking in human digestive systems. It can be accompanied by many other opportunistic and pathogenic organisms.

When one or more of these other organisms are present, successful *H pylori* therapy may not lead to any improvements in symptoms. On many occasions, *H pylori* is successfully eradicated only for symptoms to either remain unchanged or worsen and this is often because *H pylori* was only *part* of the picture.

Advantages of Comprehensive Stool Testing

On the following pages I've taken some real life stool test reports from clients who've run comprehensive testing so that you can see the level of information we're able to obtain. These tools are priceless in helping to uncover the root causes of digestive symptoms and all the complications that are caused by digestive invaders. The following three examples are extreme in that they reflect the presence of many organisms in a single person. It is not common to see so many 'bugs' in any one individual, but I often see two to three bugs in the same people when using these tests.

This is the initial stool test for a US client. You can see that the individual has *five* confirmed, positive markers for pathogenic or potentially pathogenic 'bugs'. *H pylori*, *E. coli*, yeast and fungal overgrowth, *Blastocystis* and *Endolimax nana* are all present as well as an unidentified parasite. This is an extreme case and it is rare to see this many different bugs in a single person. However, it is extremely common to see *H pylori* accompanied by other digestive invaders. Interestingly, *Blastocystis* and yeast/fungal overgrowth seem to be the most common company kept by *H pylori*. I personally had both *H pylori* and *Blastocystis*.

2100 Gastrointestinal Function Profile

Pathogenic Bacteria

Helicobacter pylori	6.6E+005 H
Clostridium difficile	<0.01
E.H.E. coli	3.1E+006 H
Campylobacter sp.	<0.01

Yeast/Fungi

Yeast/Fungi; taxonomy unavailable.	+4 => 100000 pg DNA/g specimen

A taxonomy unavailable finding may indicate ingested mold. The higher the number, the greater the indication for treatment, particularly when accompanied by clinical symptoms.

Parasites

Blastocystis hominis	Positive
Endolimax nana	Positive
Parasite present; taxonomy unavailable.	Positive

The initial test for this UK client was positive for *H pylori*. After working through *The H Pylori Diet* and stomach cleanse, the *H pylori* had been eradicated. But as you can see, there was still a significant microbial load, including *Clostridium difficile* overgrowth, *Blastocystis hominis* and *Giardia* parasites and a yeast and fungal overgrowth. The client had resolved symptoms in her upper digestive tract but she still had some 'IBS'-type symptoms in her lower digestive symptoms. The literature and clinical experience clearly shows that 'bugs' such as *Giardia, Blastocystis* and *C. Difficile* are all capable of causing fatigue, gas, bloating, pain and loose stools or diarrhoea. Subsequent phases of this client's programme were designed to help remove the parasites and restore optimal bacterial balance. This is classic example of how the root cause of 'IBS' type cases can often be uncovered with careful testing and attention.

2105 Microbial Ecology Profile

Pathogenic Bacteria

Helicobacter pylori	<0.01
E.H.E. coli	<0.01
Campylobacter sp.	<0.01
Clostridium difficile	2.8E+006 H

Yeast/Fungi

Saccharomyces sp.	+4 => 100000 pg DNA/g specimen

Parasites

Blastocystis hominis	Positive
Giardia intestinalis (lamblia)	Positive
Parasite present; taxonomy unavailable.	Positive

This stool test result shows four confirmed pathogens and an unidentified parasite. The case history for this particular client can be found at my website (see link below). As you can see, the client has *H pylori* as well as three parasites. As you will see if you read the case history, these three parasites are some of the most problematic of all the 'bugs' we find and the client's symptoms were completely consistent with those documented as being caused by these invaders. Until we ran the test, this client had been experiencing symptoms for more than a decade without ever knowing why. Read the case details at **www.H-Pylori-Symptoms.com/case-histories.**

2105 Microbial Ecology Profile

Pathogenic Bacteria

Helicobacter pylori	8.6E+005 H
Clostridium difficile	<0.01
E.H.E. coli	<0.01
Campylobacter sp.	<0.01

Yeast/Fungi

No clinically significant amounts.

Parasites

Cryptosporidium sp.	Positive
Entamoeba sp.	Positive
Necator americanus (hookworm)	Positive
Parasite present; taxonomy unavailable.	Positive

Should Your Loved Ones & Family Be Tested for *H Pylori*?

Because we are certain that *H pylori* can be passed from person-to-person I always recommend that family members are tested. Even if symptoms are not present in each member of the family, I still recommend testing. Remember that *H pylori* can happily sit in your stomach without causing obvious symptoms. Just because the symptoms are not there it doesn't mean that the bacteria are not causing damage.

If you are diagnosed with *H pylori* and you successfully eradicate your infection, it is possible that if your partner or children also have *H pylori*, they could pass it right back to you. I have seen this many times in my practice and it leads to a great deal of frustration, not to mention wasted time, money and energy. It is feasible that you may simply not be able to eradicate your infection if you are continuously being re-infected by family members.

Your *H Pylori* Testing Checklist

✓ If you are experiencing symptoms that are consistent with *H pylori*, seek testing from your doctor.

✓ If the test reveals a negative for *H pylori*, but symptoms persist, seek a second opinion.

✓ If the second test also shows a negative result, something else is likely to be causing your symptoms and a change in diet, along with a comprehensive stool analysis is recommended.

✓ If your doctor refuses to test you, see the information on stool testing at my website: **www.H-Pylori-Symptoms.com/h-pylori-testing**

✓ If you would like to shortcut this process, consider running a comprehensive stool analysis straight away so that you can identify the cause of the problem faster.

✓ If you already know you have *H pylori* but treatments are not working, or you feel worse following treatment, consider running a comprehensive stool test.

✓ If you have *H pylori*, consider having your family tested, especially if you are finding it hard to eradicate the infection or if other family members have symptoms.

✓ Always re-test at least 4 weeks after completing treatment to ensure that your infection has been successfully eradicated. Simply assuming *H pylori* infection has been eradicated because your symptoms have improved is not enough.

The importance of accurate testing cannot be over-emphasised. Your recovery depends on an accurate understanding of why your symptoms are occurring in the first place. Many of you will have the same symptoms but they may be caused by different infections and food sensitivity issues.

There's a great deal of information on comprehensive stool testing on pages 197-198. I have also posted a great deal of information on testing, including sample reports and a 60min audio recording where I discuss the testing issue in detail, at my website. Additionally, some of my clients have also been kind enough to permit me to share their case histories with you and these can be found at the website too. Go to the links below to read and listen to this great information:

Lab Testing Info:

www.H-Pylori-Symptoms.com/h-pylori-testing

Client Case Histories:

www.H-Pylori-Symptoms.com/case-histories

Why Doesn't Your Doctor Tell You All This?

Although this is a controversial talking point, I can safely say that the majority of doctors are unaware of much of the information I've presented in this book. Doctors are not *H pylori* specialists. They do a great job dealing with a huge array of symptoms on a day-to-day basis, but they are not taught about *H pylori* in detail when they attend medical school. In addition, they're so busy helping people with other ailments that they don't have time to read up to date research on *H pylori*. So the result is that they simply tend not to be aware of the latest findings.

I'd like to point out that this is not an attack on doctors. I'm merely stating the reality that I have come to know from receiving thousands of emails and phone calls from people around the world and from the very latest scientific and medical research. A huge amount of excellent research is carried out not only on *H pylori*, but also on many other common digestive infections but the findings of the research tend not to be passed down to doctors at "ground level" and so the principles highlighted in the research does not get put into practice. The following excerpt from an excellent article written by Dr. Kent Holtorf, MD, emphasises this problem:

> *"A question that is often raised by patients is "Why doesn't my doctor know all of this?" It's because the majority of physicians (endocrinologists, gastroenterologists, family practitioners, rheumatologists, etc.) do not read medical journals. Doctors do not have the time. They are too busy running their practices.*
>
> *The overwhelming majority of physicians rely on what they learned in medical school – sometimes 20-30 years ago - and on pharmaceutical sales representatives to keep them "up-to-date" on new drug information. Many studies brought to physicians for "educational purposes" are highly filtered to support their pharmaceutical product.*

There is concern from health care organizations and experts that physicians are failing to learn of new information presented in medical journals. The concern is essentially that doctors rely on what they have previously been taught and don't change treatment philosophies as new information becomes available.

This concern is particularly clear in an article published in the New England Journal of Medicine entitled Clinical Research to Clinical Practice-Lost in Translation. The author, Dr. Claude Lenfant, M.D., states there is great concern that doctors continue to rely on what they learned 20 years before and are uninformed about scientific findings. The article states that medical researchers, public officials and political leaders are increasingly concerned that very few physicians learn about new discoveries at scientific conferences and medical journals and translate this knowledge into enhanced treatments for their patients."

Did you know that it actually took Drs. Barry Marshall and Robin Warren more than *twenty years* to convince the medical establishment that *H pylori* causes ulcers? It is now self evident that *H* pylori infection causes the majority of ulcers, but for many years, Dr Marshall was ridiculed for even suggesting such a concept. I found an excellent article, written by Dr. Joseph Mercola that highlights this point:

"Truth is Violently Opposed Before It is Accepted as Self Evident"

Arthur Schopenhauer (1788-1860) was a German philosopher known for his philosophical clarity. In my view he has made one of the most valuable observations on the shifting of human views on truth as he stated that all truth goes through three steps:

1. First, it is ridiculed.

2. Second, it is violently opposed.

3. Finally, it is accepted as self-evident

This is not only true for health but all areas of life. However since my entire formal professional training is in health, I would like to share with you a dozen experiences from my professional career that validates Shopenhauer's observation, and why I will not quit despite the efforts of my critics and detractors.

Three of the 12 truths I will cover in this four-part series have reached the final stage and are now widely accepted by the medical profession, although some of my recommendations still include refinements that have yet to be embraced by conventional medicine.

The remainder is in varying degrees of acceptance, and some will not be widely accepted for quite some time, but the evidence is clear for all those who are willing to objectively review the data.

Truth # 1: Bacteria Cause Ulcers

It was 1984 when I first became aware of Helicobacter pylori (H pylori) bacteria, and its role in peptic ulcers. I learned this by reviewing the data in one of my favorite journals, Lancet. A family physician, Dr. Barry Marshall, from Australia, came up with a finding that turned the entire long held view of ulcers upside down.

I was still in my residency training when I sought to apply these findings but remember very clearly that the specialist that I reported to ridiculed me for even considering the wacky notion that bacteria could cause ulcers. I was nearly removed from my training programme for seeking to put patients on this regimen.

This was remarkable because nearly every one of the patients I put on the programme had immediate, long-lasting improvement, and did not require to go on lifelong antiulcer therapy.

When I went into private practice in 1985, the local gastroenterologists in my community considered me a renegade and would discredit me to other physicians.

Nobel Prize Awarded

However, 20 years later, in 2005, Dr. Marshall was awarded the Nobel Prize in Medicine for his discovery.

This was my first personal experience with Schopenhauer's observation.

Unfortunately, the misinformation surrounding the true cause of ulcers was still not widely known in the late '90s. A CDC survey during that time found most health care consumers were unaware that peptic ulcer disease was caused by infection with H pylori bacteria in 9 of 10 cases.

About 60 percent of respondents still believed that ulcers were caused by stress and 17 percent thought that ulcers were caused by spicy foods.

Acid Suppressing Treatments Cause More Harm Than Good

An important element of the conventional treatment of peptic ulcer disease is H2 blockers and proton pump inhibitors, which are some of the most widely prescribed drugs in the world, and there was ENORMOUS resistance from the drug companies for physicians to accept Dr. Marshall's finding.

I strongly believe that virtually all of these acid suppressing regimens are unnecessary and actually harm people. It was a major tragedy that these drugs became available over-the-counter in the '90s.

It was bad enough that physicians were using them inappropriately – now anyone can abuse these dangerous drugs and short-circuit their body's normal protective mechanisms.

Your body was not designed to have its acid level suppressed. If that occurs, then the enzymes you need to digest are not activated, and your body will not be able to fully utilise the food you eat."

So what does all this mean for you if you have *H pylori*? Well, it means that your doctor may not realise that *H pylori* is such a widespread problem. Don't be surprised if you find resistance in medical quarters when you begin to share this information with your physician. But if you do meet resistance, make sure that you refer to the evidence I've presented to you here and on my websites.

Can *H Pylori* be Eradicated?

The answer to this question is most definitely a resounding *"yes"*. H pylori can definitely be eradicated but each person's journey to freedom from symptoms will be different. I was able to eradicate my own *H pylori* infection without the use of antibiotics and I have successfully helped countless people achieve complete relief from its symptoms as well, whether it has been through referral to doctors or via the use of herbal protocols.

Antibiotic treatment and herbal programmes can both knock-out the *H pylori* bacteria. It is generally accepted that the eradication rates for *H pylori* using prescription antibiotics are somewhere between 70-75% and herbal protocols seem to work very well where antibiotics do not.

Unfortunately not everyone enjoys a smooth journey back to wellness. Antibiotic therapy does not always work and sometimes the herbal programmes need to be adjusted to suit each person's unique needs. For example, I know some of you reading this information will not be able to tolerate antibiotics such as Penicillin, whereas some of you will have great success using them. We really must consider individuality when dealing with all symptoms and metabolic imbalances.

Each of you may require a slightly different approach to successfully overcome *H pylori*:

- Some of you will eliminate all your symptoms through diet changes alone, seriously! I've seen all the symptoms of *H pylori* disappear when clients have simply eliminated simple foods from their diet. You're going to learn how to do this in the second half of this book.

- Some of you may feel, say, 50% better after changing your diet but only experience complete remission from symptoms once you have eradicated *H pylori*.

- Some of you will need to eliminate *H pylori* before you feel better at all and dietary changes may not help.

- Some of you won't feel better even if you eradicate *H pylori* because food and other infections will be causing your symptoms. Remember that *H pylori* has many cousins that can cause the same or similar symptoms.

- Some of you will feel better very quickly, but it may take a little longer for others to feel better, depending on the 'collateral damage' that the foods and infections have caused. A little healing time may be required, just as it is when you cut your finger on a piece of glass, for example.

What Is The Best Medical Treatment?

Conventional treatment of *H pylori* involves the prescription of *Triple Therapy*. Triple Therapy is based on the use of two different antibiotics to kill the *H pylori*.

Antibiotics do not work as effectively in the acid environment of the stomach, so a different type of medication is used alongside them to help reduce the acidity in the stomach. Antacid medications stop the production of acid in your stomach, which in addition to increasing the efficacy of the antibiotics, can help to relieve symptoms such as acid reflux and heartburn.

Generic names for the antacid medications often end in "zole", for example Omeprazole, Pantoprazole, Esomeprazole and Lanzoprazole. Brand names include Nexium, Protonix, Prilosec and Pantoloc. Older versions of the prescription antacids can also be found as over the counter medications in some countries, an excellent example being Prilosec. Over the counter antacid medications include Zantac (ranitidine), Tagamet (cimetidine), Rennie, Gaviscon and Tums.

Conventional triple therapy for *H pylori* usually includes one of the following combinations of antibiotics for 7-14 days. If you have taken antibiotics for *H pylori*, you will probably recognise some of these drugs. They are sometimes sold in packs such as *Prevpac* or *H Pac*:

Some example treatment options are provided in the table, below:

Option #1	Option #2	Option #3
Proton Pump Inhibitor E.g. Omeprazole, Pantoprazole Lanzoprazole, Esomeprzole **Brand names:** Prevacid, Nexium, Prilosec	**Proton Pump Inhibitor** E.g. Omeprazole, Pantoprazole Lanzoprazole **Brand names:** Prevacid, Nexium, Prilosec	**Bismuth subsalicylate**
Clarithromycin **Brand names:** Biaxin, Klaricid, Klabax, Claripen, Claridar, Fromilid, Clacid, Infex	**Clarithromycin** **Brand names:** Biaxin, Klaricid, Klabax, Claripen, Claridar, Fromilid, Clacid, Infex	**Metronidazole** **Brand names:** Flagyl
Amoxicillin **Brand names:** Amoxil, Dispermox, Trimox	**Metronidazole** **Brand names:** Flagyl	**Tetracycline** Sumycin, Terramycin, Tetracyn, Panmycin

It is accepted within the research community that the success of *H pylori* eradication treatment is declining. Resistance to the drug Clarithromycin has been shown in numerous countries to be rising to a level where the use of standard triple therapy in its current form may no longer be justified. I have read studies in which the cure rate from standard triple therapy was as low as 50%. This means that half the people who took the Triple Therapy did not eradicate *H pylori*.

It appears that the two major factors influencing resistance are prior exposure to the antibiotic and patients' compliance with therapy. Treatment regimes based on bismuth and levofloxacin are now emerging as superior protocols. Some strains of *H pylori* are more resistant to the medications than others and some of the antibiotics seem to be more effective in certain geographical regions than in others. This may account for variations in success rates seen in the literature and in practice.

In addition, it has been shown that different strains of *H pylori* can live in the same person. One strain may be susceptible to the medications but the other may be resistant. In such circumstances the antibiotics may only be effective in eradicating one of the strains.

In a 2008 report Dr. David Graham, MD, one of the world's leading medical authorities on *H pylori* wrote:

- *"Traditional triple therapy remains effective only when used to treat infections with susceptible organisms."*

- *"The prevalence of antibiotic resistance has increased to such an extent that, to maintain acceptable cure rates, all patients should be considered as having resistant infections."*

- *"Therapies that do not reliably yield 90% cure rates should not be prescribed empirically."*

- *"Triple therapies that contain combinations of a PPI, amoxicillin, clarithromycin or metronidazole now typically yield cure rates <80% and are no longer acceptable as empiric therapy."*

Sequential Therapy involves taking one antibiotic, usually for one week, followed by another for a week, whilst at the same time taking a PPI such as Nexium or Prilosec. One study showed that a group receiving sequential therapy had an eradication rate of 72.6%, versus only 58% in a group using conventional triple therapy.

Quadruple Therapy, where three antibiotics are taken alongside the proton pump inhibitor, may also be used in cases where triple therapy does not work. This strategy can involve the patient taking up to 20-25 pills per day. Some studies indicate that this method yields higher success rates whereas others show less encouraging results. In one 2007 study, for example, the success rate of using Quadruple Therapy was still only 66.7%.

Patient Screening

Because some *H pylori* strains are becoming more resistant to antibiotics, some experts have recommended that the only way to effectively manage the infection is to screen each person in order to identify the exact *H pylori* strain in each individual. Theoretically this is great concept because it enables doctors to identify whether they are dealing with resistant strains and choose eradication protocols accordingly.

The problem is that medical resources in most countries are already stretched to the limit. In some areas patients have to wait weeks or even months to even gain access to a breath test or endoscopic exam, never mind an advanced test to identify which strain of *H pylori* they may be carrying. So whilst testing for specific strains and their sensitivity to treatments would be a fantastic option, realistically this will not happen outside the research setting for a long time, if at all.

Side Effects Of *H pylori* Treatment

A strawberry or peanut can cause an allergic reaction in some people. Many people cannot tolerate eating gluten and others are intolerant to lactose. It stands to reason, therefore, that the unnatural chemical compounds that are contained in medical drugs can also cause reactions and side-effects. Dr Alan Gaby, MD, states that:

> *"Antibiotic treatment of H pylori infection is not without risk. Antibiotic therapy can lead to the development of pseudomembranous colitis, a potentially severe infection caused by Clostridium difficile. In addition, antibiotics frequently enable the overgrowth of Candida albicans, which can result in vaginitis, gastrointestinal disturbances, or other complaints. Moreover, antibiotic treatment could lead to the overgrowth of antibiotic strains of H pylori, making further attempts at eradication more difficult."*

Every medical drug comes with an information leaflet detailing the possible side effects that accompany its use. Some people don't react at all, but others can experience very unpleasant symptoms that occur directly as a result of ingesting the medication. The table below provides a summary of some of the side effects that are openly listed on the manufacturers' labels.

LISTED SIDE EFFECTS OF DRUGS COMMONLY PRESCRIBED FOR *H PYLORI*

Category Name	What it does	Drug Brand Names	Generic Names	Negative Side Effects
Antacids	Neutralizes stomach acid	Tagamet, Zantac, Mylanta, Tums, Gaviscon, Gelusil, Maalox and Rennies	Aluminium Hydroxide	Possible breast enlargement for males, dizziness, diarrhoea, fatigue and headaches
Antibiotics	Used to treat and eradicate H pylori	Achromycin, Tetracyn, Medicycline, Novatebra, Nu Tetra, Flagyl, NeoTric, Novonidazol, Trikacide, Amicillin, Novamoxin, Nu Amoxi, ProAmix	Tetracycline, Amoxicilin, Metronidazole, Clarithromycin	Possible joint pain, diarrhoea, dizziness, fever, flu-like symptoms, stomach upset, low blood pressure, kidney damage, increased liver enzymes, mouth ulcers, nausea, light sensitivity, itching, rash, skin discoloration, hives, vomiting, heartburn, shortness of breath, blood disorders and loss of appetite, Candida overgrowth

LISTED SIDE EFFECTS OF DRUGS COMMONLY PRESCRIBED FOR *H PYLORI*			
Proton Pump Inhibitors	Stops production of stomach acid. Used for treatment of Acid Reflux - GERD	Prilosec, Nexium, Prevacid, Losec, Zonton, Inhibitol, Protonix, Somac, Pantoloc, Aciphex, Pariet	Omeprazole, Lansoprazole, Rabeprazole, Esomeprazole, Pantoprozole	Possible stomach pain, constipation, diarrhoea, dizziness, upper respiratory tract infection, headache, nausea, rash, vomiting and increased risk of pneumonia
H2 Blockers	Used in Quadruple therapy to protect the stomach lining against NSAIDS. Reduces the amount of acid your stomach	Tagamet, Pepcid, Axid, Zantac	Cimetidine, Ranitidine, Famotidine, Nizatidine	Possible breast enlargement in males, diarrhoea, dizziness, fatigue, headaches, impotence and constipation.

I have received countless emails and phone calls from people who have been unable to use triple therapy because of the adverse side-effects they experience. The most common side effects seem to be:

- Fatigue

- Nausea

- Diarrhoea

- Metallic taste in the mouth

- Headaches

- Depression

- Neurological symptoms

Although antibiotics can help you heal, on the flipside they can also cause many problems. It really depends on you as an individual. I am always sad to read emails from people who had lots of side-effects when they took antibiotics for *H pylori,* only to find that the antibiotics failed to clear their infection.

The word 'antibiotic' literally means 'against life'. This is a very important point to remember. Whenever antibiotics are taken, beneficial bacteria (good bacteria that inhabit your digestive tract) that form an important and integral part of your digestive and immune systems may also be affected.

It is generally agreed that the ratio of 'good' to 'bad' bacteria needed for optimal digestion, immune function and general health, is around 85% good vs. 15% bad. When antibiotics are taken, this ratio can be altered. When this happens, the door is opened for the opportunistic overgrowth of other infectious organisms such as other bacteria – *Clostridium difficile,* for example - and yeasts such as *Candida* that can prevent recovery and even worsen symptoms.

H Pylori & Yeast/Fungal Overgrowth

A number of studies have shown that *H pylori* can survive in yeast isolated from the oral cavity. Yeast has also been found alongside *H pylori* in tissue samples taken from the stomach.

The highly acidic stomach environment usually prevents yeast from growing there and also prevents it from entering into the small intestine. Lazebnik and colleagues reported that when triple therapy was used, *Candida albicans* levels increased by 250% in *H pylori* sufferers. They also reported that *Candida* levels increased by 350% when acid-lowering medications were used on their own. The authors concluded that:

> *"The elevation of stomach pH as a result of anti-acid therapy and the elimination of H pylori with its fungicidal component from gastric mucus create optimal conditions for development of Candida in the stomach and their passage into an intestine with an early invasive growth."*

In simple terms this means that when stomach acid levels decrease as a result of *H pylori* organisms damaging the parietal cells in the stomach (the cells that produce acid) or the use of anti-acid medications, the stomach becomes more hospitable to yeast organisms. The importance of considering *Candida* overgrowth alongside *H pylori* or after treatment with antibiotics cannot be understated because if yeast and fungi overgrow in the digestive tract it can cause very similar symptoms to the *H pylori* itself.

What I'm saying here is that you can effectively eradicate *H pylori* but if you get a rebound yeast overgrowth, your symptoms could be perpetuated. I have lost count of the number of cases of yeast and fungal overgrowth that have been revealed in our comprehensive stool testing. Many of these clients were experiencing symptoms that could have been attributed to *H pylori* but their symptoms were, in fact, the result of the fungi.

Antacids Are Big Business

Whilst antibiotics can cause short term side effects, antacid medications pose a completely different problem. It is actually quite common for doctors to prescribe antacid medications to help reduce heartburn, reflux and symptoms that result from ulcers. Some people take antacids for many years, day after day. But the long term use of antacids poses several problems.

The main problem is that they shut down the production of acid in your stomach. But the acid serves two very important functions! Hydrochloric acid in the stomach is essential for assisting with the digestion of food and in particular protein. When food is inadequately digested, nutrients cannot be released and absorbed in the intestine. This is one of the reasons why *H pylori* positive patients often have low iron and vitamin B_{12} levels in their blood. Of course, iron and B_{12} are just drops in the ocean when we consider the full spectrum of nutrients required by the body, but they are the only ones that tend to be tested routinely in the medical setting. My experience has been that people who have had *H pylori* for a long time may actually develop significantly more nutritional deficiencies, which in turn cause or contribute to many symptoms, including fatigue, mood and sleep problems. Incidentally, while we are on the subject of nutrients, *H pylori* infection has been shown to reduce vitamin C levels in the stomach lining.

Digestion of food is not the only function served by stomach acid. The acid also provides a barrier that prevents unwanted organisms slipping through into the sensitive intestines. As I have already taught you, these organisms include opportunistic bacteria, parasites and yeast/fungal organisms. When stomach acid levels are too low, due to *H pylori* infection, antacids, or both, the path is cleared for these organisms to break through the barrier. This is one reason why we see so many different digestive infections alongside *H pylori* in the comprehensive testing.

Because the long term use of antacid medications compromises digestion, it has been associated with the development of serious medical conditions, with osteoporosis being the best known of these. Whilst the short term use of antacids can provide significant relief from symptoms, it should *never* be used long term in my opinion. If the root cause of heartburn symptoms is found, whether it's *H pylori*, common problem foods, low acid levels in the first place, yeast and fungal overgrowth or structural issues, the long term use of these medications is simply not required.

The Nexium 'Scandal'

In 2002, Prilosec was the third best-selling drug in the world. Prevacid, another antacid medication, was 7th in the table of best selling drugs. Apart from anything else that means that there were a lot of people walking round with heartburn and acid reflux, *thinking they needed* antacids (and there are still millions of people relying on these drugs, often unnecessarily).

Then, along came Nexium, which replaced Prilosec as the world's leading antacid drug. The way this happened deserves exposure as it constitutes an ingenius piece of deception on the part of the pharmaceutical companies and highlights everything that is wrong with the relationship between the medical and pharmaceutical systems.

As you've read, symptoms such as heartburn and acid reflux are definitely not "Nexium deficiencies" and may have several root causes:

- Hernia
- Food intolerances
- Dehydration
- *H pylori* infection
- *Candida* (or other yeast/fungal overgrowth)
- Parasites
- LOW stomach acid (often caused by *H pylori*)

Nexium is a heartburn drug of the proton pump inhibitor (PPI) type that is made by the British drug company, AstraZeneca. It came onto the market in 2001, just as the blockbuster drug Prilosec's patent was about to expire. By freaky coincidence, AstraZeneca also makes Prilosec. The company actually designed Nexium to replace Prilosec in order to protect its profits once the patent on Prilosec expired.

You may think that this sounds reasonable enough: why not create a newer, more effective product to replace an old one? This is fair enough, but once you understand the story in more detail, you'll see how it was just a big money making ploy that perhaps didn't have the best interests of the public at heart. The information you're about to read has been adapted from the work of Dr. Marcia Angell, MD.

The patenting system for drugs in the US is too complex to explain here; suffice to say that the pharmaceutical companies apply for patents on their drugs so that their competitors can't copy them. Basically, the patents give companies many years' worth of unchallenged market domination.

Once the patent expires, the door is open for other companies to produce, market and sell "generic" versions of the drugs, meaning that sales of the original drug plummet. For the public, generics are great because they are sold at much lower prices than the original drug. But for the drug companies it's disastrous.

Back in 2001, Prilosec was pulling in $6billion for AstraZeneca. If the company didn't do something quickly, its patent for Prilosec would expire and it would lose billions of dollars in revenue. Prilosec is a mixture of an active and a possibly inactive form of a molecule called *Omeprazole* (you may have been prescribed Omeprazole). What AstraZenca did is this: they took out another patent on only the active form of Omeprazole (not the inactive form). In essence, they created a new molecule that was "half of Prilosec". They then promoted this as an *improvement* on Prilosec!

Shortly before the patent on Prilosec was about to expire, the company received FDA approval for Nexium and launched an enormous advertising campaign to persuade Prilosec users and their doctors that Nexium was better.

AstraZeneca lowered the price of Nexium ever so slightly compared with Prilosec and gave discounts, free samples and any other fillip they could think of to doctors and hospitals to get them to use Nexium. They even offered coupons in newspapers. What might interest you most is that Prilosec was soon wiped from the company's advertising activities altogether. It was all about Nexium and Prilosec had essentially been forgotten. Prilosec was now being sold over the counter for a fraction of the cost of prescription Nexium.

It was basically a case of *"Buy Nexium: Half O'Prilosec for More Than Double The Price."* Mind you, they had to charge more for Nexium to cover the cost of the marketing campaign, which cost a cool $500 million to be precise in 2001. To get FDA approval for Nexium, it had to be tested in clinical trials and shown to be more effective than Prilosec. You'd think that in order to show that Nexium was better than Prilosec, they'd have run like-for-like trials, but this was not the case. Some trials compared Nexium to a placebo (a sugar pill). Not surprisingly, Nexium worked better than the sugar pills! Four clinical trials did compare Nexium to Prilosec. But oddly, these trials were done in reference to a condition called oesophageal erosion (not heartburn, which is the primary use for these drugs).

Instead of comparing equivalent doses, for example 10mg Nexium versus 10mg Prilosec, the company used *double* the dose of Nexium and the trials compared 20mg Prilosec to 40mg Nexium. You'll never guess what happened: Nexium *won*, but still only by a small margin. The logical conclusion might have been to double the dose of Prilosec rather than create a new drug, especially as people would have been able to buy it over the counter for a fraction of the cost of the prescription version. But of course, this would have lost AstraZeneca billions of dollars.

Anyway, Nexium was allowed onto the market and the rest is history. It was the third best selling drug in the US in 2005. Tom Scully, the former head of the Centers for Medicare & Medicaid Services, told a group of doctors,

"You should be embarrassed if you prescribe Nexium"

The fact that this scandalous chain of events was ever allowed to happen is one thing, but if we return to what actually causes heartburn in the first place it's blatantly obvious that antacids like Prilosec, Nexium, Prevacid, Zantac, Gaviscon are nothing more than a "band-aid" anyway. They simply do not address the root cause of the problem - they never have and they never will.

The sad thing from my perspective is that there are millions of people who have heartburn and who rely on these medications, but they are never told the reasons *why* they have their symptoms. Often, it simply takes some dietary changes to completely clear heartburn, acid reflux, stomach pain and bloating. In other cases, the patient simply needs to be tested for digestive infections such as *H pylori* and other bacteria, parasites and yeast/fungal overgrowth.

Such testing does exist and it's accessible privately to everyone, as I have already explained. Yes, it involves an investment but it's a lot cheaper to pay for a test and get rid of the underlying cause of the problem than it is to pay for heartburn medications for months and even years on end and it also reduces your risk of developing more serious conditions.

What's more, as previously mentioned, the long term use of heartburn medications unquestionably leads to other problems such as the inability to digest food and protect against parasites and fungal overgrowth. So if you have acid reflux, heartburn or any symptom that is causing you discomfort in your digestive system, first think "food" and second, think "digestive infections". Make sure you address these issues initially by following the *H Pylori Diet* and then work from there.

If you'd like to read more about how the pharmaceutical companies conduct their business, I highly recommend the book *The Truth About Drug Companies* by Dr. Marcia Angell, MD. Dr. Angell was editor in chief at *The New England Journal of Medicine* for twenty years and her detailed explanation of how drug companies deceive the public is very eye-opening.

Discontinuing Antacids

Whilst I am certainly against the long term use of antacid medications, I do not recommend that you discontinue their use without consulting with your doctor. Coming off these medications can be an uncomfortable experience. A 2010 report by the European Helicobacter Study Group, entitled *Helicobacter pylori and Nonmalignant Diseases* emphasised the importance of taking care when discontinuing antacid medications:

> *"Unselected prescription of proton-pump inhibitors in patients with dyspepsia has been questioned by the finding that withdrawal of proton-pump inhibitors induces acid-related symptoms in healthy volunteers, probably by the mechanism of rebound gastric acid hypersecretion"*

This basically means that when some people try to discontinue the PPI medications, they experience a worsening of their heartburn-like symptoms because all of a sudden their stomachs over-produce acid. I've spoken with many people who have experienced this problem. So please take care if you do make the decision to discontinue these medications and seek medical counsel prior to doing so.

Final Comment on Antacids

I recently read a good article on the BBC website, dating all the way back to the year 2000. You can read the article, below. Without going into too much detail, it suggests that antacid medications are expensive to the UK National Health Service. In fact recommendations within the article for doctors to prescribe less PPIs and at lower doses could save the UK NHS £50million worth of tax payer's money per year.

The article also mentions that running routine tests on peptic ulcer patients could place great strain on NHS testing facilities. But what about all the people out there who don't have ulcers, but still have *H pylori*? Is this an admission that it's basically impossible to screen everyone for this infection, and if so, where does that leave you if you're in the UK and you're experiencing daily symptoms?

Guidelines on indigestion and heartburn treatment could save the NHS millions, say the government advisory group behind them. The National Institute for Clinical Excellence (NICE) wants to cut the amount of an expensive indigestion drug prescribed on the health service.

But experts have warned that it may not be easy to make such pronounced savings. As many as four in ten adults suffer from symptoms of dyspepsia, or heartburn. Many of them are given high doses of drugs called Proton Pump Inhibitors (PPIs) when they visit their GPs - these are extremely effective at removing the symptoms.

However, the institute's experts argue that a great many patients would have been helped by cheaper antacid drugs, or could have had their doses of PPIs reduced with no return of symptoms. Many GPs spend more on PPIs than any other drug they prescribe, and just by cutting back in this way, millions could be saved. Patients currently on high doses can now expect these to be cut back in many cases.

Great savings

Dr Rupert Crispin, a Bognor Regis GP, said: "We've been looking at our own drug budget, and we think we could save between £30,000 and £40,000 a year this way.

"Having said that, there are a lot of other drugs coming along, such as Zyban, the smoking cessation drug, which will prove just as expensive."

However, Dr Richard Stevens, chairman of the Primary Care Society for Gastroenterology, was slightly more sceptical whether NICE's estimate of savings was achievable.

He said: "My understanding is that PPI use is still increasing at a great rate. Perhaps aiming for a decreasing rate of increase would have been more realistic."

He said: "This is a very common problem and a very effective drug."

Other parts of the guidance are likely to cost the NHS extra millions, particular advice suggesting that patients with confirmed ulcers should be tested for infection with a bacterium called H pylori.

If routinely followed, this could place NHS testing facilities under great strain.

The NICE guidance was welcomed by Health Minister John Denham. He said: "The guidance issued by NICE today means that patients can rest assured they will get the treatment that is right for them, wherever they live.

"And on top of this it will save the NHS money - as much as £50 million a year."

While it is not compulsory that NICE guidance be followed to the letter, it is likely that GPs will attempt to observe restrictions on PPI use, in order to save money on their drug budgets.

Read this article online at:
news.bbc.co.uk/1/hi/health/829125.stm

In my opinion, whilst some of you - whichever country you are in – will doubtless receive the medical care you need and deserve, many of you will become very frustrated with the lack of appropriate understanding, testing facilities and the budgetary restrictions imposed on insurance companies and health services. This was one of the main drivers behind me writing this book. I want you to know that alternatives to conventional healthcare are available if you know where to look. You most certainly can access the appropriate tests and expertise to enable you to restore balance to your health.

Natural Health Alternatives

I am walking proof that *H pylori* can be eradicated using a natural programme. A number of foods and herbs have been scientifically and clinically proven to work against *H pylori* but it's important to understand that the studies are often performed in a lab dish or test tube and not in a human body. The results of these studies and the spurious claims from supplement manufacturers that accompany them must be taken with caution.

Because I've seen it happen so many times over the last three years, I can guarantee 100% that some of you reading this will experience a complete recovery from your symptoms by changing key aspects of your diet alone. Unfortunately, some of you may not experience improvements using diet changes and you may also need to add medical treatment or use a herbal protocol to restore a favourable balance of bacteria in your digestive system.

Some of you will need to check for other digestive infections because, as I have alluded to several times, *H pylori* has 'partners in crime' such as yeast overgrowth or parasites such as, *Blastocystis hominis, Giardia* and *Cryptosporidium.* Even when diet changes are made and *H pylori* has been eradicated, symptoms can continue if these other 'bugs' are not cleared. But with due diligence, you can overcome your symptoms relatively quickly and without experiencing the side-effects that conventional treatment can cause.

Summary of Section One

I've taught you how *H pylori* causes obvious symptoms and how it can also be very 'sneaky' and potentially contribute to a whole host of seemingly unrelated symptoms and diseases.

We know that *H pylori* infection increases the risk of developing ulcers and more complex digestive symptoms, as well as being associated with anaemia, skin disorders, fatigue, depression, sexual dysfunction and sleep problems. Although the precise mechanisms of action are not known, many of these symptoms probably result from nutritional deficiencies and the wider effects of chronic stomach and intestinal inflammation.

We also understand that *H pylori* is the number one risk factor for certain stomach cancers. Recent research has focused on the role of *H pylori* in creating metabolic imbalances that lead to insulin resistance, diabetes, heart disease and stroke.

Unfortunately, we know that doctors' knowledge of these problems is not consistent, which leads to problems in accessing the right testing and treatments. Even when the correct diagnosis is made, treatments do not always work and may cause side effects. Even when treatments do successfully eradicate *H pylori* there is no guarantee that symptoms will improve unless diet changes and other digestive imbalances are addressed.

The good news is that just like countless people before you, you have the ability to bypass all this confusion and uncertainty. Part Two of *The H Pylori Diet* is going to provide you with a programme that has been shown time and time again to safely and effectively restore the correct balance to your digestive system and remove the unpleasant symptoms that you have been experiencing.

So it's time to get moving with your *H Pylori Diet* action plan!

Part Two - Featuring *The H Pylori Diet*

Introduction to *The H Pylori Diet*

Working on a one-to-one basis with my clients on a daily basis affords me the luxury of understanding each person's health history and circumstances in great detail. In writing a book, I am unable to derive such detail about you.

Each of you is a unique individual with a completely unique set of symptoms and life circumstances. Whilst I have done my very best to include as much information as I possibly can in order to help you overcome your *H pylori* symptoms, I cannot make outrageous guarantees that you will do so using the information in this book alone.

I run my practice and write my books with the highest level of honesty and integrity and what I *can* guarantee is that if you follow this programme step-by-step, you will feel much better *unless* you have hidden and unidentified factors that act as road blocks to your progress.

Many of your chronic symptoms will clear as you eliminate simple foods that cause inflammation in your stomach and intestine, improve your sleeping patterns and learn to control your blood sugar levels. You will have more energy, begin to gravitate towards your optimal weight, enjoy better sleep and relax into more stable and uplifting moods.

The H Pylori Diet guide provides the foundation for your success and, at your discretion, may be supported on a clinical level by laboratory testing and specific supplement protocols to help balance and boost the different systems of your body that are in need of support.

Whilst the majority of you will have great success using this programme, some of you may need additional resources and support in the form of laboratory testing and specific protocols to help clear the road blocks.

No Magic Bullet

If you want to successfully eradicate *H pylori* and then, importantly, keep it away, it is *vital* to understand that there is no magic bullet cure. If you have *H pylori*, there will often be other issues that you need to address in order to elevate your health to your desired level. I'd like to provide you with an example of what I mean.

I actually discovered that I had *H pylori* while I was working with Dr. Dan Kalish, a chiropractor and Functional Medicine practitioner of some fifteen years. I actually spent six months on Dr. Kalish's Functional Medicine internship, learning how to apply natural medicine so that I could help my clients heal faster. At the time, I had some nasty heartburn and reflux symptoms, so I ran a stool antigen test, which returned positive for *H pylori*. After running a natural stomach cleanse, my symptoms disappeared and I felt much better.

However I soon developed diarrhoea, which was very unusual for me. I ran a retest, using the same stool antigen test procedure. It came back negative for *H pylori*, which was great news because it meant that the programme had worked, but it showed up a positive for a parasite called *Blastocystis hominis*. 'Blasto', as I affectionately call it, is a relatively common human parasite and can be the underlying cause of so-called Irritable Bowel Syndrome (IBS). When I ran a separate herbal protocol to eradicate the parasite, my loose stools disappeared.

My point is that *H pylori* may not be the only factor contributing to your symptoms. In many cases, *H pylori* can be successfully eradicated but symptoms remain, or new ones appear. In these cases, it is important to do further investigation in order to uncover the cause of the problem. Food sensitivities can play a huge role creating your symptoms, which is why careful consideration of diet is so important.

Unfortunately many people – including doctors - believe that taking a bunch of antibiotics or herbs to kill *H pylori* is a panacea and will solve all problems. This is simply not the case because if the infection has been present for many years and there is damage to your digestive system, your body will need time to heal from any 'collateral damage'. Remember that the metabolic imbalances that are caused by chronic inflammation can be widespread. If there is a lot of collateral damage, your symptoms may take some months to resolve.

It is my goal to not only help you overcome *H pylori* but to also teach you sound nutrition and lifestyle principles that will help you prevent re-infection and remain at the pinnacle of your health for many years to come. I want to help you make your body bullet-proof so that it becomes difficult for anything to get in there and start causing problems!

Some of you will find this programme easy to apply and some may find it more challenging. You will need to eliminate certain foods to reduce inflammation in your digestive system, eat health-giving foods to support your body's own innate healing power, sleep enough to allow your immune system to do its job and remove as much stress as you possibly can from your life. It is important to understand that adhering to these recommendations is a critical factor in determining your success. You can take the best, most expensive supplements in the world, but if you do not provide a solid foundation for your healing, the supplements simply may not work.

Using The *H Pylori Diet*

Please take the time to read through *The H Pylori Diet* guidelines in full and then choose the aspects of your diet and lifestyle that are going to be easiest to change first. If you feel that you cannot implement all the changes immediately, please do not worry. Take the programme step-by-step. Just imagine what you can achieve in ten weeks by changing just one aspect of your diet and lifestyle each week.

I strongly encourage you to eliminate gluten, cow's milk and soy from your diet as soon as you possibly can. These are, perhaps, the most important steps in the entire process. I have seen people's symptoms clear *completely* by taking these steps alone.

The supplement recommendations provided in the stomach cleanse section of the programme are based on many years of clinical experience and teachings that have been passed down to me by number of leading natural health practitioners.

As I have found new ways of helping my clients, I've adapted these protocols to suite the legal requirements of different countries. Different protocols exist, for example, if you live in Australia.

If your symptoms are mild, I recommend waiting *at least 8 weeks* from commencing the nutrition programme before you use the supplement protocols. However if you are in discomfort, using the supplements immediately may bring significant relief from your symptoms. In the unlikely event of your symptoms not improving, or if you would like to significantly accelerate your progress, I strongly recommend that you take advantage of our personalised consultancy services as your case may require additional evaluations and expertise.

Simply send an email to **Office@HPExperts.com** and my office staff will respond to your enquiry within 24 hours. Details of our services and full contact details can be found on page 197-202.

Finally, I welcome and encourage your comments, feedback and success stories. We must constantly strive to improve our educational materials to benefit you, so we actively encourage you to send feedback and suggestions on how we may improve our service.

Understanding Your Digestive System

Before I teach you how to overcome *H pylori* and its associated symptoms, it is extremely important for you to fully understand and appreciate the basics of how your digestive system works and how *H pylori*, other digestive infections and food intolerances can affect your digestive system's ability to do its job properly.

In so doing you will see precisely why it is so important to adjust your diet and lifestyle so that you optimise digestive function.

The Three Roles of Your Digestive System

Your digestive system has three primary roles, the optimisation of which are absolutely essential for you to regain and maintain optimal health. Simply put, if your digestive system is not working properly, it is *impossible* to have optimal health.

- First, your digestive system breaks down food into its constituent nutrients so that your body is able to absorb them.

- Second, it has a defensive role, protecting your body against potentially dangerous particles and organisms that enter in the air, food and water to which you are exposed. These particles include bacteria such as *H pylori* and *Salmonella*, viruses, parasites like *Blastocystis* and *Giardia lamblia*, potentially toxic chemicals in the air, food and water, moulds, dust and many others.

- Third, it acts as a waste disposal unit, helping you to eliminate toxic substances from your body. These include toxins in the environment, waste products from your body's own metabolism and the unused portions of the foods you eat.

Digestion from the Top Down

Your digestive system is essentially a tube leading from your
mouth to your anus. The entire system includes other organs,
such as the pancreas, liver and gallbladder, which squirt liquids
into the digestive tubing to help service specific needs in the
digestive process. The "digestive tubing" itself has several
names and you will commonly see it referred to as one of the
following:

- Alimentary canal
- Gastrointestinal tract, or GI tract
- Digestive tract
- Gut

The GI tract is roughly 26 feet, or 8 metres long. It is divided
into a number of distinct sections:

Mouth

Your mouth is more important than you may think! It is the
first stage of the digestive process. Chewing breaks up food
into manageable lumps. The food also mixes with saliva,
which lubricates the movement of the food down your throat
and oesophagus and also helps to begin the breakdown of
carbohydrates and fats through the action of two enzymes:
salivary amylase and lingual lipase.

In these days of busy, stressful lifestyles, it is common to see
people bolt down their food without chewing it properly.
If you do not chew your food adequately, the first stage of
digestion is not completed thoroughly and this may lead to
a 'domino' or knock-on effect on digestion further down
the tube. My favourite digestive test, the *GI Effects* test from
a laboratory called Metametrix, shows how well my clients
are digesting fats, proteins and vegetable matter in addition
to spotting 'bad' bugs. If the test shows that they are not
digesting their food properly, I encourage them to chew
thoroughly when they eat!

Throat & Oesophagus

When you swallow, food is directed down your oesophagus, towards your stomach. The oesophagus is a muscular tube and under normal circumstances it squeezes food down towards the stomach with waves of muscular contraction known as peristalsis. Food reaches your stomach around 6-8 seconds after you have swallowed it.

Stomach

The stomach is a 'J'-shaped bag. It has a heavily folded lining (the folds are called *rugae*). It is separated into three sections: the *fundus* at the top, *body* in the middle and *antrum* at the bottom. *H pylori* bacteria tend to live in the antrum, close to the *pylorus*, or *pyloric valve*, which acts like a trapdoor between your stomach and small intestine.

Your stomach is very muscular, which enables it to churn and mix food, much like a washing machine rotates to effectively wash your clothes. Food is mixed with digestive enzymes and hydrochloric acid to produce a soupy substance called chyme, which passes into the small intestine, where the digestive process continues.

Small Intestine

Around 80% of nutrient absorption occurs in your small intestine. The small intestine is around 8m/20ft in length and is divided into three sections, the *duodenum, jejunum* and *ileum*.

The *duodenum* is the first and shortest section of the small intestine, averaging about 25cm in length. It acts like a mixing bowl, blending juices from your liver, gallbladder and pancreas with the soupy chyme from your stomach.

The jejunum is usually around 2-2.5m/7-8ft long. The majority of nutrient absorption occurs through this section of the intestine. Fats and sugars are absorbed into your body in the duodenum and jejenum. If you are unable to absorb these nutrients properly, they may reach the colon in an undigested state, causing gas, bloating and sometimes diarrhoea.

Minerals such as calcium, iron and zinc are also absorbed here, as are the water soluble vitamins – most B vitamins and vitamin C - and the fat-soluble vitamins A, D, E, K and folic acid.

More digestion and absorption occurs in the *ileum*, which is the longest section of the small intestine at around 3.5m/11-12ft. The ileum is the only site where vitamin B_{12} can be absorbed into your body.

Intestines Are Amazing Structures

The lining of your intestines is not flat. It is a highly specialised environment consisting of numerous different cells and structures. *Villi* are finger-like projections that stick out from the lining of the small intestine. *Each of these villi is covered in* tiny hairs, called *microvilli*. These structures help to significantly increase the surface area, making the absorption of nutrients much more efficient. They are sometimes known as the *brush border*.

Between the villi are structures known as the *Crypts of Lieberkuhn*. You will read more about these crypts later. They become deeper when there is inflammation in the intestines, providing an ideal hiding place for bacteria and parasites.

Please refer to the *H Pylori Diet* e-book for colour diagrams that accompany these descriptions!
See **www.H-pylori-Symptoms.com/e-book**

Goblet cells line the crypts and villi. Their job is to secrete mucus to protect the delicate intestinal lining against particles and chemicals that could potentially cause damage.

Enterocytes also line the villi and crypts. On the villi, these cells are responsible for absorbing nutrients – vitamins, minerals, amino acids, fatty, acids, sugars – from the chyme.

Large Intestine (Colon)

The main function of your large intestine, or colon, is to absorb water. As the remains of your food are pushed through the colon, around 2 litres of water are absorbed. The longer it takes to expel faecal matter, as in constipation, the greater the amount of water absorbed and the harder it can be to eliminate the waste.

Your colon is also inhabited by trillions of 'friendly' bacteria that digest fibre and other particles of food. In fact, there are more bacteria in your digestive tract than there are cells in your body. Approximately one third of faecal matter is bacteria! Many of these bacteria are also beneficial because they help to make certain vitamins, such as some B vitamins and vitamin K. They also keep unwanted bacteria, yeasts and parasites in check.

Three other organs supply the digestive system with essential fluids and chemicals that are essential in the digestive process:

The Liver

Your liver is an amazingly versatile organ and is responsible for many functions. In fact, scientists believe that the liver has more than four hundred different functions. As a digestive organ, the liver makes *bile*, which contains salts that help to neutralise the acidic chyme as it enters the small intestine from your stomach. The salts also help to break up large molecules of fat into tiny ones so that they can be digested and absorbed properly through by the villi.

The Gallbladder

The gallbladder acts as a storage tank for bile that has been made in your liver. In the gallbladder, water is removed from the bile, making it up to twenty times more concentrated. Bile is squirted into the duodenum when it is needed for the digestive process. Interestingly, *Helicobacter* species have been isolated in both the gallbladder and the liver and it is believed that they may contribute to significant problems in those areas, most notably the development of gallstones.

The Pancreas

The pancreas produces a fluid called *pancreatic juice* that contains a number of important enzymes to help break down food. The fluid is also alkaline, helping to neutralise the acidic chyme as it enters into the intestine from the stomach. You may be interested to know that several studies have shown an association of *H pylori* infection to pancreatitis.

The Impact of *H Pylori* on Your Digestive System

It is important that you understand how your digestive system works so that the recommendations I make throughout this book make sense for you. Anything that compromises the function of your digestive system has the potential to cause health problems and jeopardise your healing process.

How Does *H Pylori* Damage Your Stomach?

Once it is in your stomach and intestine, *H pylori* can cause an inflammatory response that damages the cells lining the stomach. The *parietal cells* that are responsible for producing stomach acid may become damaged. Research indicates that *H pylori* bacteria prime the immune system to make antibodies that actually attack the lining of the stomach and, in particular, the parietal cells that make acid.

This condition, where your own immune system begins to attack its own tissues, is called an *autoimmune* reaction. The autoimmune attack against the parietal cells can lead to a reduction in the production of stomach acid. Once stomach acid is low, it is not possible for you to digest and absorb food properly. This can lead to:

• A slow passage of food through the digestive tract.

- Symptoms such as heartburn, bloating, constipation and abdominal pain.

- Nutrient deficiencies such as iron deficiency (anaemia) and B-vitamin insufficiency.

If stomach acid levels are too low, food may sit in your stomach for too long and putrefy. The gases produced during this putrefaction can cause reflux, heartburn and other unpleasant symptoms. The biggest problem with this scenario is that doctors will often prescribe heartburn or reflux medications because they think the symptoms are being caused by *too much* acid. Here, treatment using anti-acid medications often exacerbates the problem! Interestingly, studies have shown that *H pylori* bacteria prefer to live in the *least* acidic areas of the stomach. It is therefore possible that antacid and PPI medications such as omeprazole and lanzoprazole may actually help *H pylori* survive.

Gastritis & Ulcers

H pylori bacteria penetrate and attach themselves to the outermost layer of the stomach lining. Ammonia gas produced by *H pylori* is toxic to cells and can cause direct damage to the lining of your stomach and small intestine. Some strains of *H pylori* have a protein called *Cytotoxin Association Gene-A, or* CagA. These strains are strongly associated with ulcer formation and stomach cancer and seem to be the most important strains in the studies that have found associations between *H pylori* and heart disease.

CagA strains physically inject a toxin into the mucosal lining using a syringe-like structure called a pilus. CagA damages the lining of the stomach by separating the joins – known as tight junctions - between stomach cells.

Certain strains of *H pylori* can also make a protein called VacA, which attaches to stomach lining cells, creating holes or bubbles inside the cells (called vacuoles). Eventually this process can also damage the stomach lining cells.

Once these processes have begun, your immune system begins to send immune cells to the scene of the damage. The sudden influx of immune cells causes the tissue in your stomach lining to rapidly inflame, just as your finger would if you hit it with a hammer. The immune cells release very powerful chemical weapons to fight the *H pylori*; however, in the fight between the immune cells and *H pylori* an appreciable amount of damage to the stomach lining occurs. The resulting stomach inflammation is known as *gastritis*.

Once chronic gastritis sets in, the repeated insults to the stomach lining cause degradation and destruction of the cells. This can eventually lead to a condition called *atrophic gastritis*. Interestingly, research suggests that *H pylori* tends to disappear – like a vanishing act - once the gut reaches this level of damage. It's as though the bacteria can no longer live in the stomach once they have damaged it to this extent.

Ulcers can also develop in your stomach or small intestine as a result of the ongoing irritation and inflammatory response. They can be very deep and may even eat through the entire thickness of the stomach or intestinal wall. Ulcers can also occur close to blood vessels, resulting in blood spilling into the stomach or intestinal cavity.

> *Remember, if you are in severe pain, passing blood in your stools or vomit, have dark, tarry stools or vomit containing dark granules, you should see a doctor immediately as you may have a bleeding ulcer.*

Secondary Infections

If *H pylori* organisms have damaged your digestive system and compromised acid and enzyme levels in your stomach, you may also acquire what I call a *secondary infection*. Stomach acid not only helps you to digest food, but also helps to kill parasites, opportunistic bacteria, moulds and fungi that enter your digestive system in food and water. If your stomach acid and enzyme levels are low, it is much easier for these invaders to pass through and colonise the lower areas of your digestive tract.

The most common digestive invaders I see are *Candida albicans* (yeast/fungal), *Blastocystis hominis, Giardia lamblia, Cryptosporidium* and bacterial overgrowth such as *E. coli, Pseudomonas and Yersinia*. I have even seen *Salmonella, Vibrio* (which can cause cholera) and several types of worm infections, including whipworm, pinworm, threadworm and hookworm. I highly recommend that you see the Case Histories page at my website to see real life test reports. You may like to check for these bugs using a comprehensive stool antigen test should your symptoms do not clear on this programme.

Case Histories:

www.H-Pylori-Symptoms.com/case-histories

Information on Stool Testing:

www.H-Pylori-Symptoms.com/h-pylori-testing

H Pylori and the Gallbladder

I was very interested to discover that *H pylori* and other *Helicobacter* species have been isolated in the gallbladder because I had already made the observation that many of my clients with *H pylori* also had at some time had their gallbladders surgically removed. Studies do indicate that *Helicobacter* infection of the gallbladder may lead to a greater risk for gallstone formation. I strongly suspect that *H pylori* may be responsible for many gallbladder surgeries and that testing for *H pylori* in these circumstances may reduce the need for such invasive and unpleasant experiences. If you have gallbladder problems or gallstones, I recommend that you ask doctor to test for *H pylori* and seriously consider adopting some diet and lifestyle changes.

The *H Pylori* Diet

Now you know exactly what *H pylori* is, the symptoms it causes, how to test for it and how it damages your digestive system, it is time to learn how to reduce your symptoms with *The H Pylori Diet* and run a special *Stomach Cleanse* that should help to remove the bacteria from your system.

Phase One of the process is the foundational nutrition and lifestyle system that I recommend to all my clients. I cannot stress the importance of this phase of the programme enough. Some of my clients have experienced incredible results with the foundational programme alone. You will learn why the programme can lead to such dramatic improvements as you read on.

Phase Two contains the Stomach Cleanse that many people have used with great success to restore normal microbial balance in their digestive systems. The Stomach Cleanse teaches you how to use the most effective supplements, in the optimal amounts, for the right length of time and in the correct sequence.

Take This Programme at Your Own Pace

The H Pylori Diet contains a series of recommendations for you to add into your daily schedule. I do not want you to feel overwhelmed by the information so I suggest that you read through it at least once and make notes on the recommendations that are going to be easiest for you to implement. The one thing that I ask is that you pay special attention to *removing certain key foods* from your diet, namely cow's milk, gluten and soy.

I have provided you with food lists, meal ideas and useful resources but it is important that you make the effort to find the best food sources in your area. You may be reading this book in Australia, South Africa, the UK, North America, New Zealand, Hong Kong or any other country and it's impossible for me to provide resources for you in all these different locations.

Once you have read through the information at least once, start by eliminating the key foods as detailed at the start of the programme, one by one, or all at once if you feel this is possible. You may be surprised by the improvements these simple changes bring.

Once you have successfully eliminated these foods, focus on including more of the appropriate foods that I have listed. When writing a book of this nature, it is very hard to cater for individual preferences. However at this point I'd like to recommend that you check out the comprehensive recipe book that was written by my colleague, Karen Maidment. Having experienced *H pylori* and parasite infections herself, Karen put together a complete book of recipes that compliment my recommendations perfectly. You can find details of the *H Pylori & Digest-Ease Recipe and Cookbook* at the web page, below:

www.H-Pylori-Symptoms.com/recipe-book

Some of the key diet recommendations presented in the *H Pylori Diet* may surprise you and we do receive emails from customers who are a little overwhelmed with the amount of information presented in the *H Pylori Diet*. If you do feel a little confused about where to start, please see details of our Health Freedom Secrets programme on pages 199-201. This programme is designed specifically to help you implement the programme step-by-step.

The Stomach Cleanse

I recommend that you follow the nutrition and lifestyle programme for approximately 60-days before running the stomach cleanse. This will help to reduce inflammation in your digestive system so that the supplements are more effective. Continue to adhere to the nutrition and lifestyle recommendations during and after the stomach cleanse.

Of course, if your symptoms are severe and you feel that you must try to take herbs to work against *H pylori* as soon as possible, you can begin the stomach cleanse immediately. In this scenario it is still very important for you to follow the nutrition and lifestyle portion of the programme as closely as possible.

How Quickly Will You See Results?

This is the perennial question asked by my clients and in the many email correspondences I receive and if I knew the answer then I truly would be a guru! The answer is, genuinely, "*I do not know*". I don't know because you are all unique individuals and will have your own set of symptoms and circumstances.

Some of you will experience excellent results very quickly by omitting certain foods from your diet. Many of you will see gradual improvements as the weeks go by and will feel much better after the stomach cleanse. A proportion of you may be disappointed by your progress and this usually indicates that other factors – for example nutritional deficiencies, other digestive infections or food allergies – are contributing to your symptoms. The good news is that I have provided information and resources to help you uncover these roadblocks.

"I felt compelled to make contact with you after following your advice on diet. I have had several doses of anti-biotics for my helicobacter and although I may get relief for a short time it always comes back. I have my energy back, I have no pain, no nausea I feel more confident. I just cannot believe it. I am eternally grateful to you for the well researched advice. You have given me my life back." **Anne, Glasgow, UK.**

The *H Pylori* Diet Phase I - Foods To Avoid

Step One – Eliminate Gluten

"From your advice I have now been gluten free for only the past 3 weeks, and I have already seen a massive difference in my health. I have finally been able to stop taking Omeprazole (a drug I have now been on since May 07, and thought I would have to continue taking for the rest of my life). I generally feel happier, lighter, free from aching joints, etc. Although I'm not completely better, this is a good start, and I know I have many changes yet to make, and many habits yet to break" **MP, Lancaster, England.**

Avoiding gluten is possibly the single most important step you can take towards wellness.

What is Gluten?

Gluten is a protein molecule found in many common grains, especially wheat, barley and rye. Because many convenience foods are grain based – for example pasta, bread, crackers, cakes, biscuits - people are exposed to gluten on a regular basis. In fact, gluten-containing foods are the mainstay of the western diet, which as you'll see causes a huge problem. Gluten is also in the majority of processed and packaged foods as well as alcoholic beverages such as beer.

What Is The Problem?

If you have digestive symptoms, there is a very good chance that you're what we call *gluten-intolerant*. When you eat gluten, the gluten protein molecules may be causing inflammation and an immune reaction in your small intestine. The reaction damages and flattens the intestinal villi. Remember that the villi are finger-like projections in the lining of your intestines and are essential structures for helping you to absorb vitamins, minerals, sugar, amino acids, fats and oils into your body. Over time, eating gluten can seriously damage your intestines and lead to poor absorption of nutrients. This progression can be seen below:

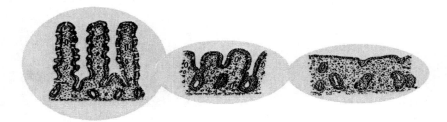

Healthy villi   **Partial atrophy of villi**   **Total atrophy of villi**

If you are gluten sensitive, you will almost certainly develop nutritional deficiencies. For example, studies have shown that gluten sensitivity and *H pylori* infection can both cause anaemia due to the inability to absorb iron and vitamin B_{12}. Other B vitamins such as B_1, B_2, B_5, B_6, folic acid and lipoic acid often become depleted. These vitamins are essential for energy production, detoxification, brain function and many other aspects of a healthy physiology.

Symptoms of Gluten Sensitivity

I'd like to make it absolutely clear that gluten sensitivity can cause the same or similar symptoms as *H pylori*. If you are gluten-sensitive you will typically experience heartburn, bloating, diarrhoea, constipation, mind fog, headaches, fatigue, skin conditions, depression and anxiety. In fact, the overlap of symptoms is so vast that people with *H pylori* may experience a near 100% improvement in symptoms *simply by removing gluten from their diet*. Gluten sensitivity really is a hidden plague.

"Dave

I gave up gluten 16 days ago. The improvement in how I felt was almost instant. I feel like a different person. I also quit taking my Prilosec. Right now I'm regular, no bloating or any intestinal problem and all my other body aches and pains went away. I appreciate what I've learned so far.

All the best, Mark"

The most severe form of gluten-sensitivity is a condition called Coeliac disease (spelled 'celiac' outside the UK). Coeliac disease usually involves significant reactions to gluten that can induce severe pain with blood and mucus in stools and diarrhoea. However a cohort of Coeliac patients does not tend experience acute digestive symptoms. Instead, people in this cohort may feel fatigued, anxious or depressed, experience weight loss, anaemia and may not even be diagnosed with Coeliac disease until they have bone scans that reveal osteoporosis. In many ways, gluten-sensitivity is insidious and causes hidden damage in the same way as *H pylori* does. Just because the consumption of gluten is causing repeated damage to the gut, it doesn't mean that you necessarily feel or sense that damage when you consume the gluten.

One of my favourite doctors, Tom O'Bryan DC, is a staunch advocate of gluten-free living and on his website he quotes some startling statistics about the symptoms of gluten sensitivity:

- 73% of Coeliac patients have clinically diagnosed Trait Anxiety Disorder and 63% have Depression (American Journal of Medicine Volume 116, March 1, 2004)

- All children clinically diagnosed with ADHD or their parents report a significant improvement in their behaviour and functioning after 6 months on a gluten-free diet (Journal of Attention Disorders, March 2006, 1-5)

- 70% of unrelenting migraines were completely relieved on a gluten-free diet (Neurology, Vol. 56/No. 3, Feb.13, 2001),

- In young adults with unrecognised, silent Gluten Intolerance, scholastic attainment and professional underachievement was 400% more likely (Scan.J.Gast ro,2005;40:1407-1412)

- 50% of children with drug-resistant epilepsy successfully achieve remission on a gluten-free diet (Lancet 1992 Aug 22;340(8817):439-43).

It is possible that some – or many - of your symptoms are being caused by gluten sensitivity so you may benefit significantly from removing gluten from your diet. Some people notice improvements in the way they feel within days. For others, noticing the benefits of a gluten-free diet may take longer because the gut lining will need time to heal.

Gluten is Addictive

For some of you, avoiding gluten will be very challenging. Gluten is in plenty of commonly eaten foods. Any food made with wheat, rye, spelt or barley contains gluten. So bread, pizzas, breakfast cereals, crackers, biscuits, pasta, beer, lager and other common foods and beverages should be avoided. Gluten is also used as a thickener in many canned, processed and packaged foods. But don't panic because convenient and delicious alternatives are all part of the programme!

When you first eliminate gluten, some of you may experience cravings - of varying intensities - for gluten-containing foods. If you are gluten-sensitive, addictive chemicals are produced by your body when you eat the foods. These chemicals are called gluteomorphins and are chemically similar to heroin and morphine. Wikipedia states that:

Gliadorphin (also known as gluteomorphin) is an opioid peptide that is formed during digestion of the gliadin component of the gluten protein. It is usually broken down into amino acids by digestion enzymes. It has been hypothesized that children with autism have abnormal leakage from the gut of this compound, which then passes into the brain and disrupts brain function.

If gluten sensitive people do not eat gluten for a few hours, a drop in gluteomorphin levels can trigger another craving or induce feelings of depression or anxiety. This is like the 'comedown' from drug-taking and can be a powerful addictive agent. Some people also refer to this pattern as 'comfort eating'. Just think about the common 'comfort foods' for a moment: if they don't contain a lot of sugar, they usually contain gluten!

Possible Withdrawal Symptoms

During the initial days or weeks of eliminating gluten you may suffer withdrawal and other physical symptoms, including headaches, nausea, tremors, difficulty sleeping, depression and irritability. You may also experience cravings for other foods such as caffeine and sugar. On the other hand, you may stop eating gluten and feel great immediately – it really depends on your reaction as a unique individual.

One of the tools I use to assess how addicted my clients are to gluten is to check their reaction when I tell them they need to stop eating it. The more they object, the more likely they are to be gluten intolerant. It's like a drug addict being told to give up his or her drug of choice. If you feel like you would miss gluten or don't know what you would do without it, then you could well be addicted to it.

Inflammation from gluten reactions in the intestines typically takes 60-days or more to subside and then the gut lining can take a further three months to a year to heal completely. However healing times may be much longer in cases where gluten sensitivity is severe.

"Good Grains"

I recommend that you consume moderate helpings of the following grains because they do not contain the harmful gluten molecules:

✓ Rice	✓ Quinoa
✓ Buckwheat	✓ Teff
✓ Millet	✓ Amaranth
✓ Corn/Maize	

Pastry, pasta, bread, crackers, cakes, biscuits and most other processed foods contain gluten. Beers and many spirits also contain gluten as they are made from grains. Use rice cakes, corn crackers, gluten-free pasta and bread as replacements for these foods. If you must consume alcohol, drink very small amounts of wine or distilled spirits and *never* drink on an empty stomach.

"Bad Grains"

To be safe, *avoid* any food that is made from or has the following ingredients:

✗ Wheat (including flour)	✗ Barley
✗ Rye	✗ Spelt
✗ Oats*	✗ Semolina
✗ Couscous	✗ Beer, lager, most spirits

Be careful to avoid ingredients such as 'modified starch', as they most probably contain gluten. The safest and simplest way to avoid gluten is to eat a natural, whole food diet that does not contain any processed foods.

*Oats do not contain gluten but they may be refined in the same factories, so if you do eat oats please ensure that they are definitely processed away from gluten grains.

Non-Gluten Food Replacements:

Pasta: you can buy gluten-free pasta made from rice, buckwheat, corn and millet.

Bread: health food stores often stock gluten-free bread. **Rice bread** is a favourite of mine. You can also use **rice** or **corn crackers**.

Baking: If you enjoy baking, there are gluten free alternatives to wheat flour: **Coconut flour, arrowroot flour** and **rice flour** can all be used. You can find many recipes on the Internet that use these types of flour.

Beers & Spirits: Wine & cider are alternative alcoholic drinks but you should always remember that alcohol is a toxin to the body in any form or amount, causing cortisol levels to rise and stress on your liver.

If you would like to learn how to create lots of delicious recipes using these alternative ingredients I highly recommend that you order the *H Pylori Digest-Ease Cookbook* that's available at

www.H-Pylori-Symptoms.com/recipe-book

How Much Gluten Can You Tolerate?

It has been shown that as little as one eighth of a teaspoon of wheat flour is enough to cause an inflammatory reaction in gluten-sensitive people. I highly recommend, therefore, that you try to eliminate gluten foods from your diet completely. You must become a *Food Label Detective*. Check all food labels to make sure they do not contain gluten.

Step Two – Eliminate Processed Cow's Milk Foods

As you have already learned, if you have *H pylori*, you may also be gluten sensitive. If this is the case, you possibly also have a cow's milk intolerance. Inflammation caused by gluten-sensitivity and/or digestive infections damages the cells in your intestine. If the cells that produce the enzyme *lactase* are damaged, you will no longer be able to digest the *lactose* sugar molecules that are found in cow's milk.

Symptoms of lactose intolerance can be similar to those caused by gluten sensitivity and *H pylori:* bloating, wind, diarrhoea and abdominal pain. Even *without* gluten intolerance, some people are simply lactose intolerant anyway and cannot digest cow's milk products. Others still may react to a substance called *casein*, which is one of the proteins found in cow's milk. Some people react to the protein, some will react to the lactose. Some unlucky people may react to both.

As your intestinal lining heals on a gluten-free diet you may be able to tolerate cow's milk products again within 60-90 days, but you should certainly seek to omit both gluten and all cow's milk products for an absolute minimum of 60-days. You can then introduce them again and see whether they cause your symptoms to return or worsen.

Lactose Intolerance Home Test

There is a simple home 'challenge' test for lactose intolerance and while this test *may not reveal every case of lactose intolerance* it may help you to identify whether cow's milk is contributing to your symptoms.

Avoid milk products for one week. Upon awakening drink a large glass (8-12 oz.) of whole milk on a completely empty stomach. Do not eat or drink anything else for 3 to 4 hours. If you experience bloating, gas, diarrhoea, abdominal discomfort, mucous in the throat or abnormal bowel habits, you are likely to be lactose intolerant. In some cases the symptoms may not appear immediately, but should be noticeable within 24 hours.

If you experience no reaction whatsoever, you <u>may</u> not be lactose intolerant. However it is also important to remember that you may be allergic to the casein proteins in milk, even if you are not lactose intolerant and that this test may not reveal that casein reactions.

Not All Milk Is Created Equal

Only a small percentage of cow's milk products in the Western world are consumed raw. Raw milk is, for many people, a health-promoting food. It is packed with nutrients that help the immune system and provides an abundance of healthy vitamins, minerals and friendly bacteria such as *Lactobacillus*.

Pasteurised and homogenised milk, however, are not healthy foods. Unfortunately most of the dairy products we consume as a society are pasteurised. Pasteurisation radically alters the structure of proteins in milk and destroys many of its beneficial nutrients, including the good bacteria that are necessary for keeping your digestive and immune systems healthy.

In addition to this, much of the milk produced in commercial farming is of a poor quality because the cows are fed low grade grain foods and even road-kill. In the US, cattle are also fed hormones and antibiotics, the residues of which build up in the cow's body and are passed to humans via beef and milk.

Cows are designed to eat grass, not the grain products and soy that they are fed through modern, commercial agriculture. If you drink milk or eat cheese and butter that has come from an unhealthy animal, you will most likely not be healthy yourself.

Buying Raw Milk

When you do reintroduce cow's milk after 60-days, aim to drink high-quality, raw milk from local farmers who look after their herds properly. Many people who are unable to tolerate pasteurised milk can tolerate raw dairy products. A wonderful resource for you to explore is **www.realmilk.com**. You will find a wealth of useful information on this website, including a list of producers and suppliers. Readers in the UK will also enjoy the website **www.seedsofhealth.co.uk**, which lists a number of raw milk suppliers. Explore local farmers' markets and cow share programmes as you will doubtless find some excellent suppliers of raw milk products in your area.

Use Goat & Sheep Milk

Goat and sheep's milk tends to be more compatible with human physiology and if you are having trouble weaning yourself away from all milk, they can be great replacement options for you. Alternatively, try using a little rice milk or almond milk.

If you would like to read more about the controversy surrounding the dairy industry, read the work of Robert Cohen. Robert has written two very controversial books entitled *Milk: The Deadly Poison* and *Milk A-Z*. You may also wish to visit **www.mercola.com** and type 'milk' into the search engine. You will find numerous interesting articles on milk at this site.

In my comprehensive ten-week *Health Freedom Secrets* programme, we go into a little more detail about both gluten and cow's milk, including the specific ways in which they cause health challenges and a more detailed discussion on how to make sure you can easily implement gluten and milk-free living into your lifestyle.

Step Three – Avoid Soy

If you eat large amounts of soy-based products, it is certainly in your best interests to cut right down on soy or eliminate it from your diet completely. Some years ago, when I was trying to find the best solution for people who wanted to lose weight, I'm ashamed to say I was promoting soy-based protein shakes. I was also drinking these shakes myself. I continually had digestive problems such as flatulence and loose stools. It didn't take me long to realise that whenever I stopped using the shakes, my digestion returned to normal. When some of my clients began to experience similar problems I knew for sure that the soy protein was a major problem. Gluten and cow's milk don't seem to affect me as much as they do others, but soy is something I just can't tolerate!

Soy has been touted as a health food for a number of years. However it is becoming a serious problem. Many people react to soy just as they do to gluten. In fact, if you are sensitive to milk or gluten, there's a high chance that you may be reacting to soy as well because these foods all contain protein molecules that can irritate the gut lining.

In *The Whole Soy Story: Dark Side of America's Favourite Health Food*, Dr. Kayla Daniel states:

> *"Thousands of studies link soy to malnutrition, digestive distress, immune-system breakdown, thyroid dysfunction, cognitive decline, problems, reproductive disorders and infertility - even cancer and heart disease".*

I do not want to bore you with the whole story of how soy has become so popular. If you would like further information, read Dr. Kayla Daniel's book and review the articles on soy at **www.westonaprice.org**.

Soy, like gluten, is found in about two-thirds of processed and packaged foods. It is very important to put the packet down if the ingredients list has the words 'soy' or 'soya' on it, but as you can see below, there are other, hidden sources of soy that you should be aware of.

For example:

- Tofu
- Soy milk
- Soy infant formula
- Soy protein isolate
- Soybean oil
- Soy protein concentrate
- Soy lecithin
- Texturised or hydrolised vegetable protein (hidden sources of soy)

Good Soy?

If you would like to eat small amounts of soy from time to time, choose fermented soy products such as tempeh, miso, natto, soy sauce and tamari. Eat small amounts of these foods and gauge whether your symptoms are aggravated in any way.

Step Four – Cut Back on Your Sugar Intake

Sugar Encourages Yeast Overgrowth

Some people take antibiotics for *H pylori* only to feel much worse than they did before they started. If you recall some of the previous information in this book, you'll know that the use of both antibiotics and PPI medications such as Nexium are associated with the overgrowth of yeast and fungal organisms such as *Candida*. The overgrowth of these organisms can cause a huge variety of symptoms. This is one reason why people may feel the same or even worse after completing a course of antibiotics. I like to teach my clients that their symptoms are usually a combination of three main factors:

1. *H pylori*
2. *Other infections*
3. *Food*

In other words, there's something in there that shouldn't be! If you have athlete's foot, vaginal or oral thrush, jock itch, dandruff, a white/yellow coated tongue, burning mouth, eczema, brain fog or sweet and bread cravings, you likely have a digestive yeast infection that demands attention.

Eliminating the problem foods, as discussed in this section and clearing your *H pylori* and yeast infections will almost certainly help you to feel much better. *Candida* thrives on sugar so it is very important to minimise sugar and other processed carbohydrates – bread, pasta, cookies, cakes, etc – in order to keep the *Candida* under control.

Sugar Compromises Your Immune System

Sugar has been shown to reduce immune function within minutes of its consumption. As I have mentioned several times already, you need your immune system to be functioning as effectively as possible in order to overcome *H pylori* and keep it away. Complete avoidance of sugar isn't always necessary, but the majority of people benefit from reducing its consumption significantly.

Avoiding Sugar

Just as it can be quite hard to avoid gluten, processed milk and soy, so too can it be difficult to avoid sugar. Again, trying to adhere to a natural, whole food diet automatically helps you to avoid these problem-causing foods. Some sources of sugar are obvious, like table sugar, for example. However there are some hidden sources of sugar that you need to be aware of. Be wary of labels that contain the words that end in 'ose':

- **Dextrose**
- **Lactose**
- **Galactose**
- **Sucrose**
- **Maltose**
- **High-fructose corn syrup**

Soft Drinks

Soda-pop drinks as well as sports drinks should also be avoided. Coke, lemonade and other fizzy drinks can contain as many as 8-12 teaspoons of sugar per can. These drinks are a serious threat to your health and can contribute to obesity, depression, skin problems blood sugar problems such as hypoglycaemia and diabetes. They have also been implicated in osteoporosis and dental problems.

Fruit

Even the sugar contained in fruit and fruit juice can cause problems. You may not realise that the commercially bought fruit juices are actually not much more than 'sugar juices'. Indeed, an eight-ounce glass of fruit juice contains around eight teaspoons of sugar. Because the juice is not bound up with fibre as it would be in the actual fruit, it causes problems with blood sugar handling in the body. I do not recommend drinking store-bought fruit juices at all. If you are going to take fruit juice, purchase a fruit and vegetable juicer and do the juicing yourself. A little further on we explore the benefits of juicing in more detail.

Step Five – Throw Out The Bad Fats

Much of the nutrition information we are given by the media, physicians and education system is questionable. The reason for this is that it is based on what the food manufacturers want you to believe so that they can sell their highly processed products and make billions of dollars in the process. We explore this topic in greater details in the *Health Freedom Secrets* online programme.

High quality fat is your *friend*. It is especially important for you to eat high quality fats and oils because the intestinal damage caused to the intestine by gluten sensitivity and digestive infections destroys structures in the villi called lacteals. It is the lacteals that help you to absorb fatty acids from the fats and oils you eat. People who have suffered with digestive complaints for a long time will typically be deficient in certain fatty acids. A key step in your quest for overcoming *H pylori* is to learn which fats are good for you and which ones are doing you harm. I have no doubt that some of you will be surprised to learn that high quality fat is probably not the type of fat you imagine.

Good Fats

✓ Animal fats (as long as they are from healthy animals)

✓ Olive oil

✓ Flax oil (unheated, very small amounts)

✓ Coconut cream, milk & oil

✓ Raw cow's, goats and sheep dairy

✓ Nuts & seeds (seasonal and in small amounts)

✓ Raw nut butters (e.g. almonds, cashews)

✓ Olives

✓ Avocados (small amounts)

✓ Egg Yolks (& whole eggs)

Bad Fats
(if consumed in high quantities)

All vegetable, seed and nut oils including these commonly used oils:

✗ Sunflower oil

✗ Safflower Oil

✗ Peanut Oil

✗ Soy Oil

✗ Avocado Oil

✗ Walnut Oil

✗ Corn Oil

✗ Cottonseed Oil

✗ Sesame Oil

✗ Canola Oil

✗ Margarine and all 'butter substitutes'

✗ Hydrogenated fats

✗ Partially hydrogenated fats

Contrary to popular belief, research shows that excess vegetable oils are not good for you as they are very sensitive to heat, oxygen and light. They degrade very easily and become difficult for your body to process. In fact, the oxidation of these oils in your body can be a cancer risk, a topic that is discussed in detail in the research of Dr. Ray Peat at **www.RayPeat.com**. It is *not* my intention in this book to enter into a detailed discussion on this topic, but I highly recommend that you read some of Dr. Peat's articles for further information and evidence and, as previously mentioned, this topic is discussed in greater detail in my *Health Freedom Secrets* programme.

Cooking In Fats & Oils

The only fats and oils you should cook with are:

✓ **Coconut Oil**

✓ **Butter (after 60-days of avoidance)**

✓ **Ghee (after 60-days of avoidance)**

✓ **Lard (ideally from organically raised, healthy animals)**

Ideally you should only cook with animal fats and coconut oil. The other vegetable oils – even olive oil – are prone to damage at high temperatures. If you do choose to use olive oil, add it to your dish towards the end of the cooking process so that it is not exposed to high heat for too long.

An added benefit of coconut oil is that it is an antimicrobial agent. Coconuts contain lauric and caprylic acids, which can damage unfriendly bacteria, yeasts and parasites. In fact, monolaurin is used by many practitioners to help reduce *H* pylori infections. The medium chain fatty acids in coconut oil are also excellent sources of energy that your body can readily utilise.

Eating The Right Fat Does Not Make You Fat!

There is a lot of misinformation surrounding fat. Historical evidence shows that heart attacks, high cholesterol and other conditions did not increase until we started to eat commercial produced vegetable oils, margarines and high volumes of sugar.

Many of the health problems we see today actually result from the consumption of sugar, processed oils and plastic butter-like products that are sold as margarine. According to leading expert Dr. Mary Enig, vegetable oil spreads on the store shelves look more like plastic than anything in Mother Nature's pantry when they are examined under a microscope.

Dr. Diana Schwarzbein, a world-renowned diabetes specialist, discusses in her excellent books the fact that eating fat is not the main factor in most people gaining weight. In fact, it is the over consumption of carbohydrates and sugars that causes weight gain. If you eat too much carbohydrate and the body's stores become full, your body has no alternative but to convert the sugar into fats and cholesterol in the liver. In fact, Dr Schwarzbein argues that the body has no mechanism for storing fat *unless* carbohydrates and sugars are consumed!

If you are worried that eating saturated fat may elevate your cholesterol levels, I urge you to read Justin Smith's book *29 Billion Reasons to Lie About Cholesterol* in which he presents a wealth of medical and scientific evidence, showing that:

- The body's primary source of cholesterol is that which is made in the liver.

- A high sugar diet is the primary dietary cause of high cholesterol.

- Eating fat and cholesterol does not elevate cholesterol levels.

- Statin drugs are ineffective in preventing heart attacks.

When you combine this with the excellent information presented on Ray Peat's website and the practical information I cover here and in *Health Freedom Secrets*, you'll soon realise that you have nothing to fear and everything to gain by consuming healthy fats and oils.

Be a Fat Label Detective

If you see the following words on a food label, avoid them. If these ingredients are in processed and packaged foods, they will already be rancid and toxic:

- **Vegetable oil**
- **Hydrogenated vegetable oil**
- **Partially hydrogenated vegetable oil**
- **Soy oil**
- **Peanut oil**
- **Safflower oil**
- **Sunflower oil**

Phase One – Review

Try to avoid these key foods

✗ Gluten-containing foods
Replace them with rice, millet, buckwheat & corn products.

✗ Pasteurised Dairy Products
Avoid as much as possible; switch to goat and sheep products.

✗ Soy, including tofu, soy protein shakes and all soy foods
Except some fermented soy products – tempeh, miso, natto, small quantities of soy sauce.

✗ Sugar (including fruit juices and soft drinks)

✗ Vegetable Oils and Margarines

Other Potentially Problematic Foods

In addition to the main foods I have already discussed, you may find that the following foods aggravate your stomach:

Alcohol

Strangely, some studies have actually shown that alcohol can suppress *H pylori*. However, alcohol is not a good option when you have *H pylori*. Alcohol damages the lining of your digestive system and can seriously aggravate your condition. Alcohol will play havoc with your blood sugar and lower immune function. If you do not avoid alcohol for three-four months during your attempt to clear *H pylori*, the programme may not work. The odd glass of wine with a meal is OK, but it is best to aim for total abstinence if possible. You should certainly never drink on an empty stomach.

Vinegar and Condiments, including tomato ketchup and other sauces

The acidity in these may aggravate the lining of your digestive system and can cause pain and burning. It is best to limit these foods during your programme. Malt vinegar contains gluten as it is derived from barley.

Pickled Foods

Again, the acidity in the pickles can aggravate the lining of the stomach.

Smoked & Salty Foods

Smoked foods are generally not healthy choices. The salt and curing processes can lead to aggravation of the stomach lining and these foods have been linked to cancer.

Phase Two – Eat More Good Foods

How To Use The *H Pylori Diet* Food Guide

1. I have tried to make the Food Guide as easy for you to follow as possible. Here are the basic guidelines:

2. The **bold black** foods are your **primary foods**. Eat them freely.

3. The foods in *italics* are *secondary foods*. Eat them occasionally, in small amounts, or as supplementary foods to the primary ones.

4. Include a primary protein food at each meal (meat, poultry, fish or seafood).

5. Include two or more vegetables at each meal.

6. Add fruit, goat/sheep dairy, eggs, oils and fats as desired.

7. *Add Secondary foods in italics* to provide variation, flavouring and dressings as desired.

8. **If it is not on the list don't eat it!** You'll see that foods such as bread, pasta, cakes, cow's milk, cheese, soy, tofu, alcoholic beverages and certain oils (e.g. canola oil) are not listed. I have omitted all gluten, cow's milk and soy-containing foods. I have also omitted all foods that contain refined sugar.

9. Foods that are high in starchy carbohydrate and sugar have been omitted or placed in italics to help you with blood sugar balance.

10. If this appears to be a little complicated, please read on as the practical guidelines on how to implement the foods list are presented shortly. Also, don't forget to check out the *H Pylori Digest-Ease Recipe and Cookbook*, written by my colleague and qualified chef, Karen Maidment.

Meat & Poultry		Fish & Seafood	
Beef	Chicken (dark meat)	Abalone	Oysters
Buffalo	Chicken (white meat)	Anchovy	Perch
Elk	Cornish Hen	Bass (freshwater)	Pompano
Heart (beef)	Duck	Bass (sea)	Rockfish
Kidney (beef)	Goose	Catfish	Roughy
Lamb	Pheasant	Caviar	Salmon
Liver (lamb / beef)	Quail	Clams	Sardine
Pork (bacon)	Turkey (dark meat)	Cod	Scallop
Pork (ham, chops)	Turkey (white meat)	Crab	Shrimp
Rabbit		Crayfish	Snapper Squid
Venison		Grouper	Trout
		Halibut	Whitefish
		Herring	Shark
		Lobster	Swordfish
		Mackerel	Tuna
		Mahi-mahi	
		Mussels	
		Octopus	

Legumes	Beverages	Dairy and Eggs	
Aduki Beans	Tea (herbal)	Feta	Eggs, Chicken (whites)
Black Beans	Vegetable Juices	Goat Cheese	
Black-eyed Peas	Water (pure, filtered)	Goats Milk	Eggs, Chicken (yolks)
Broad Beans	Tea (black)	Goats Yoghurt	Eggs, Duck (whole)
Butter Beans	Coffee (caffeinated)	Goats Butter	
Chickpeas	Coffee (decaf)	Sheep Milk	
Great Northern Beans		Sheep Cheese	***ALL PRODUCE
Green Beans	Not more than one cup of	Sheep Yoghurt	SHOULD BE
Green Peas	coffee or tea per day and		FREE-RANGE OR
Kidney Beans	always drink in morning		ORGANIC WHERE
Lentils	Fruit Juices (freshly		POSSIBLE***
Mung Beans	squeezed, not bought in		
Navy Beans	store)		
Pink Beans	Oat Milk		
Pinto Beans	Rice Milk		
White Beans	Almond Milk		

Nuts and Seeds		Greens	
Almonds	*Pecans*	**Beetroot Greens**	**Lettuce (round)**
Brazil Nuts	*Pine Nuts*	**Chard**	**Mustard Greens**
Cashews	*Pistachios*	**Coriander**	**Radicchio**
Chestnuts	*Poppy Seeds*	**Dandelion Greens**	**Rocket**
Filberts	*Pumpkin Seeds*	**Endive**	**Spinach**
Hickory Nuts	*Sesame Seeds*	**Kale**	**Spring Greens**
Macadamia Nuts	*Sunflower Seeds*	**Lettuce (iceberg)**	**Sprouts (alfalfa)**
Peanuts	*Walnuts*	**Lettuce (loose-leaf)**	**Sprouts (bean)**
		Lettuce (romaine)	**Turnip Greens**
			Watercress

Vegetables			Sea Vegetables
Artichoke	Daikon (asian radish)	Tomato	Agar
Asparagus	Fennel	Water Chestnuts	Dulse
Aubergine	Garlic	*Butternut Squash*	Irish Moss
Avocado	Ginger Root	*Parsnip*	Kelp
Bamboo Shoots	Jerusalem Artichoke	*Pepper (hot, all*	Laver
Beetroot	Jicama	*colors)*	Wakame
Bok Choy	Kohlrabi	*Potato (all varieties)*	
Broccoli	Leek	*Pumpkin*	
Brussels Sprout	Mushroom (all varieties)	*Squash (summer)*	***ALL PRODUCE
Cabbage	Okra	*Swede*	SHOULD BE FREE-RANGE
Carrot	Olive (all varieties) Onion	*Sweet Potato (yam)*	OR ORGANIC WHERE
Cauliflower	Pepper (bell, all colors)	*Sweetcorn*	POSSIBLE***
Celery	Radish	*Turnip*	
Courgette / Zucchini	Shallot		
Cucumber			

Fruits			Oils and Fats	
Apples	Grapes	Persimmon	Goats Butter (unsalted)	*Evening Primrose Oil*
Apricots	Guava	Pineapple	Coconut Oil	*Hemp Oil*
Banana	Honeydew	Plums	Fish Oil	*Sesame Oil*
Blackberries	Melon	Pomegranate	Olive Oil	*Sunflower Oil*
Blueberries	Kiwifruit	Raspberries	*Almond Oil*	
Boysenberries	Kumquat	Rhubarb	*Black Currant Oil*	
Cantaloupe	Lemons	Strawberries	*Borage Oil*	
Casaba	Limes	Tangerines		
Melon	Loganberries	Watermelon		
Cherries	Mango			
Coconut	Nectarines	*Currants*		
Cranberries	Oranges	*Dates*		
Elderberries	Papaya	*Figs*		
Gooseberries	Peaches	*Prunes*		
Grapefruit	Pears	*Raisins*		

Herbs, Spices and Seasonings		Grains
Anise	Mace	Amaranth
Basil	Marjoram	Buckwheat
Bay Leaf	Mustard	Millet
Caraway	Mustard Seed	Oat
Cardamom	Nutmeg	Quinoa
Cayenne	Oregano	Rice (brown)
Chervil	Paprika	Wild Rice
Chilli Powder	Parsley	
Chive	Pepper (ground	
Cinnamon	black) Peppermint	
Cloves	Rosemary	
Coriander	Saffron	
Cumin	Sage	
Curry Powder	Salt (sea salt,	
Dill	unrefined)	
Fennel Seed	Savory	
Fenugreek	Spearmint	
Garlic Powder	Tarragon	
Ginger	Thyme	
Horseradish	Turmeric	
	Vanilla (extract)	

Vinegar (apple cider)	Chocolate (dark)	
Vinegar (balsamic)	Honey	
Vinegar (rice)	Ketchup	
Vinegar (wine)	Mayonnaise	
Wasabi	Molasses	
Carob	Sugar (brown,	
	unrefined)	

***ALL PRODUCE SHOULD
BE FREE-RANGE OR ORGANIC
WHERE POSSIBLE***

Meal/Recipe and Planning Ideas

I appreciate that it can be difficult to change your diet, especially when you have been eating many of the foods that I am recommending you avoid! I've listed some simple meal ideas for you that are completely gluten, milk and soy-free and that are also low in sugar and 'bad' fats. I am also very happy to admit to you that despite possessing a good working knowledge of functional nutrition, I am no chef!

If you feel that the resources within the book are limited and you'd like a lot more variation in the meals and recipes you use, please do go online and get the *H Pylori Digest-Ease Recipe & Cook Book*, written by my colleague and qualified chef, Karen Maidment. The book can be ordered at **www.H-Pylori-Symptoms.com/recipe-book**.

Breakfast

It is important to view breakfast as just another meal. Unfortunately social conditioning leads us to believe that breakfast has to consist of specific foods such as cereal, toast, croissants, orange juice and fruit. Many of these foods are based on cereals, which contain gluten and are mostly consumed with cow's milk! The truth is that your body simply wants high quality nutrients and it is fine to eat *any* healthy food for breakfast! I hope it doesn't sound patronising, but moving away from social stereotypes is an important step forward if you want to regain and maintain optimal health.

If you have a light appetite:

- Boiled egg with gluten-free bread, toasted and an apple.

- 1-2 slices of ham with corn crackers, hummus and an orange.

- Soft Goats cheese, rice cakes and a piece of fruit.

- Healthy Smoothie - see the smoothie recipes at **www.H-Pylori-Symptoms.com/smoothies**

If you have a stronger appetite:

- Smoked salmon, small avocado, olives and add some salad – spinach, lettuce, tomato, etc.

- Smoked mackerel fillets, small avocado, finished with some berries.

- Grilled nitrate-free bacon (not overdone), eggs (yolks cooked) and small glass of fresh vegetable/fruit juice to finish.

- Chicken or turkey salad (white and dark meat) – green lettuce, celery, tomato, parsley, scallion/spring onion. Dressing – olive oil (can mix olive oil with apple cider or balsamic vinegar)

- Last night's leftovers (a tactic I use with many clients, leftovers provide an easy, nutritious meal!)

Breakfasts can be finished with an apple or pear slathered in raw nut butter (hazelnut, peanut or cashew butter). Make sure the nut butter is raw, or made with *unroasted* nuts. Cooking nuts damages the delicate oils and makes them susceptible to damage.

Lunch

- Sliced roast beef, grated or sliced goats cheese, mixed lettuce, peppers, onions, mushrooms, olive oil dressing with apple cider vinegar*.

- Smoked salmon with lettuce, tomatoes, cucumber, avocado and olives, dressing of olive oil on its own or with apple cider vinegar + herbs.

- Celery sticks wrapped in ham or other roast meat slices Dip into raw soured cream flavoured with dill or chives

- Steak with lettuce, tomato, onion, cucumber

- Roast chicken leg, salad of spinach, olives, avocado, tomato

- You may add 2-3 rice or corn cakes (spread raw nut butter if desired) to any meal.

- Last night's leftovers!

- Fruit dipped/slathered in raw nut butter can be used as a dessert

Note: do not use apple cider vinegar until any stomach pain, burning or bloating has disappeared. Do not exceed 1tbsp of apple cider vinegar.

Dinner

- Steak & egg with avocado, peppers, onions mushrooms and olive oil/herb dressing.

- Chicken thigh with steamed broccoli, kale, leek and cauliflower.

- Salmon fillets, vegetables, goat's cheese salad.

- Thai soup or curry containing chicken or prawns.

- Familiar meals such as chicken/turkey and vegetable soup, chilli con carne, Thai curry dishes, stews and hotpots are all excellent choices. Add plenty of vegetables

- With these meals, small baked potatoes with lots of raw goat's butter, goats cheese or some wild/brown rice with lots of olive oil can be eaten in moderation.

Note: don't eat large quantities of starches with your meals: small servings such as a small potato, or 2-3 new potatoes, a handful of carrots or half a cup of rice, are fine. Eating too many starchy foods at the same time as protein-based foods can be stressful to your digestive system.

Food Quality & Shopping Tips

Buy Organic

Although it is usually more expensive, organic produce is more nutritious and contains fewer harmful chemicals than commercially raised/grown food. When I say 'more expensive' I would like to clarify that in supermarkets, organically labelled food tends to be more expensive than non-organic, or commercially raised food. I have my doubts regarding the labelled foods in supermarkets and I must admit that I feel the 'organic' label is being used as a sales tool in a lot of places.

However, it is possible to acquire fresh produce of superb quality at local farmers markets and co-ops. Because you buy direct from the farmer the prices are generally much more reasonable than the equivalent 'organic' supermarket foods. The farmers may not have an organic logo to put on their produce, but they generally operate with integrity and a genuine love and passion for what they produce. Go out of your way to buy fresh, in season and locally grown food where possible rather than shopping at the supermarkets. If you buy food at the supermarket, even if it says 'organic' on the label, it may not be as nutritious as locally grown, fresh food that doesn't carry the logo.

Look for butchers, farmer's markets or cooperatives in your area. Talk to the farmers and get a feel for how passionate they are about their produce and work. You will find that the smaller-scale, local farmers care deeply about the quality of the food they sell. You will not get the same passion at a supermarket because the supermarkets compete on price, not quality. Using a farmer's market or a good butcher usually removes a link in the financial retail chain. This makes purchasing your high quality foods much less expensive.

I highly recommend that you also research organic food delivery services on the Internet. There are many delivery companies that specialise in sourcing fresh, whole and organic food in many countries. Shop around and find one that you like.

If you do need to shop at the supermarket, only shop round the edges/perimeter of the store. You will find the aisles are stacked with processed and packaged foods, but the fresh produce is almost always around the perimeter.

> The food itself should be the only ingredient and it should not need a label. Apples, steak, salmon and carrots do not need ingredient labels telling you what is in them!

Do Not Fall For Clever Marketing

"Organic" or "Natural" on the label does not mean "Healthy". Organic sugar, pasteurised milk and white flour are not healthy, even if they are marketed as organically grown. This is one of my pet peeves. There is no doubt in my mind that companies are exploiting food labelling laws in combination with the organic movement. Some foods are just not good for you, it doesn't matter whether they are 'organic' or not.

The more a product is advertised, the less healthy it is. Think of Coca-cola and Mars Bars. Some of the most destructive foods are those that just happen to be advertised most. You do not need to advertise good food – it advertises itself.

Frozen & Tinned Food

Try not to buy frozen food. Buy your food fresh and if you think you may not use it, or you want some food in the freezer to fall back on, freeze your freshly purchased foods. Freezing causes foods to lose nutritional value, but home-freezing of fresh food can be convenient. Frozen food is better than tinned food, although I admit to keeping a stock of organic tinned tomatoes in my cupboard.

Meat

Buy the leanest cuts of meat, especially if you are unable to find organic or free range meats. Toxins are stored mainly in fatty areas of the body. When an animal consumes toxins, they are stored in the fat because most toxins are what we call fat-soluble. If you then eat the animal fat, you also get a dose of toxins.

This doesn't apply so much to animals that are fed a natural diet and kept in optimal living conditions. These animals will generally be much healthier and happier! Cows that live in barns all their lives and chickens that are caged in disgusting battery farms should be avoided completely.

Poultry & Eggs

A recent U.K government survey showed that organic laying hen farms have significantly lower levels of *Salmonella*. The study showed that 23.4 per cent of farms with caged hens tested positive for *Salmonella* compared to only 4.4 per cent in organic flocks and 6.5 per cent in free-range flocks.

Eggs laid by free range hens have also been shown to contain less saturated fat and cholesterol and more vitamin A, omega-3 fatty acids, vitamin E and beta-carotene, than commercially laid eggs. The message is this: go out of your way to avoid battery hens! The birds do not see the light of day, live in tiny cages and eat foods that they were never designed to eat, including their own shit!

Seafood

When you buy seafood, try to buy smaller species of wild, coldwater fish: sardines, herring, mackerel, sea-bass are good examples. Almost all seafood is now contaminated with mercury. The further up the food chain you go, the higher the levels of mercury are. This means that fish such as shark, marlin, salmon and tuna contain high levels of mercury.

Try to avoid farmed fish as they tend to harbour the highest concentrations of toxic metals. You will also see, for example, that the flesh of farmed salmon contains much bigger fatty streaks in their meat than that of wild Alaskan or sockeye salmon.

My *Health Freedom Secrets* programme contains interviews with some of the world's leading experts on these topics. They are absolutely critical topics to understand. The programme is available at a significant discount to you – fifty per cent, to be precise - as a valued reader of this book.

Tips for Busy Lifestyles

Adopting the dietary changes I have outlined takes some planning. In fact, busy modern lifestyles are the number one reason in my experience why people find it tough to implement the recommendations. It is certainly possible for you to make all the changes I have suggested by taking care to plan your meals. You have the resources and technology at your fingertips to get on top of time constraints and there really is no excuse not to eat healthily if you embrace the tips listed below.

Cook in Large Batches

Go out of your way to cook *too much food*! Cooking large batches of food or meals will ensure that you have food left over for the next day. For this purpose I highly recommend the book "*Real Foods, Real Fast*", by Rico Caveglia, as long as you avoid the gluten-containing grains.

Use Leftovers!

One of the ways I manage to have a healthy breakfast is to eat the leftovers of my previous night's meal. This is a far healthier way to start the day than eating processed, fast food like cereals, toast, croissants, pancakes or doughnuts. Leftovers are also great to come home to after a busy day's work when you "can't be bothered" cooking a meal from scratch! Almost anything you cook can be stored and used to make a meal the next day. You can also freeze the food you cook for future use if the batch is large enough.

Eat More Raw Food

The more raw food you eat, the less time you will need for preparation. Eating raw foods not only cuts down preparation time but also ensures that sensitive nutrients in the food are not destroyed in the cooking process. Foods that can be eaten raw include vegetables such as celery, carrots, tomatoes, cauliflower, radish, onion, scallion/spring onion, seeds, nuts, berries and unpasteurised dairy. If you are eating meat, you can also cut down on preparation time by eating them rare-medium as opposed to well done where applicable.

Prepare Tomorrow's Meals Today

When you are at work and lunch comes round you will probably have a hard time finding good quality food on the high street. At the time of writing, I live in London and if I don't prepare my lunch the day or night before, I can struggle to find healthy options. Most of the available options in the city canteens, stores and cafes contain processed food, bread, cheese, low quality vegetables and are generally not particularly appetising.

It is much easier, less stressful and healthier to pick up your lunch from the refrigerator before you leave home rather than making it in the morning, so I highly recommend preparing tomorrow's lunch today. Again, you may use leftovers from previous meals or prepare a healthy salad that will only take around 5-10min to put together the night before.

Eat Nutritious Foods

This might sound obvious, but the higher the quality of food you eat, the less you will *need* to eat. Food serves a purpose: to provide as much healthy nutrition as possible to help you deal with the stresses of your day to day activities, heal your body and help you grow and repair.

If you want to heal, have more energy and save time, eat fresh, whole, organic food that provides the nutrients your body needs rather than processed foods that may appear filling, but actually only provide empty calories (calories devoid of any vitamins and minerals).

In *Health Freedom Secrets*, one of the most important lessons teaches you about the 'Life Force' of foods. The more processed the foods are, the less life force they contain so that when you eat them, they actually take more energy out of your body during the course of digesting and eliminating them than they give back. It's no wonder so many people feel tired!

Know Your Dinner Before You Leave The House!

If you leave your house in the morning knowing what you are having for dinner that night you will feel more relaxed about time. You can either cook something that is in the refrigerator on your return, heat up leftovers or pull something out of the freezer before you leave home. Being organised in this way ensures that you will not need to fall back on unhealthy convenience or junk food, microwave meals or takeaways.

Know What You're Buying

If you plan your meals properly, you will know exactly what you need to buy when you go grocery shopping. This will help you economise and will minimise the chances of you wasting food and, therefore, money. Plan to shop twice per week – once every 3-4 days – so that you only eat fresh food and please take advantage of our recipe and meal resources in other publications.

Use a Food Delivery Service

Using a food delivery service can be a godsend if you are struggling to find time to do a proper shop. You will find many companies that provide a delivery service for high quality, organic and free range produce. These companies can usually deliver on a specified day or even morning / afternoon when you know you are going to be in to collect the delivery. If you are out at work all week, ask a neighbour, local store or friend to take the delivery for you. Payment is usually taken at the point of order so the groceries can be delivered to your specified address without the need for payment on delivery.

Preparing Your Food

Cooking needn't be complicated. Even if you are an inexperienced cook, preparing uncontaminated, healthy food can be made easy by following some basic principles.

- Ensure that you have a good vegetable juicer so that you can quickly juice vegetables that provide high levels of vitamins and minerals. Continue reading for my juicing guidelines.

- Go out of your way to buy a good blender so that you can mix eggs, raw dairy products – milk, cream, yogurt etc. – nuts, oils, protein powders, coconut milk, fruit, etc. into your vegetable juice to make smoothies.

- If at all possible, buy a juicer and blender for work as well and keep fresh produce in the refrigerator there. Even better, ask your employer to buy one for you!

- Don't cook using any vegetable oils. Only use coconut oil or raw butter or add olive oil at the end of the cooking process.

- Experiment with herbs and spices to add fuller flavour to your food and make it more enjoyable. Try to buy organic herbs to avoid pesticide exposure and be very careful with spices such as cayenne and chilli as they may irritate your stomach.

- Keep vegetables fresh by squeezing as much air out of the vegetable bags as possible. This can actually increase the 'shelf-life' of your vegetables by 2-3 days.

- It is important to thoroughly wash food - especially fruit and vegetables – before eating. Using plain old tap water may not wash the food properly and this can lead to parasitic infection and the ingestion of chemicals that may be harmful and add to your stress load. Remember that the food you eat should help your body deal with stress, not add to it!

- You can clean your food by letting it sit in water and 4-8oz distilled vinegar for 30min. This is especially useful if you are using non-organic produce as it will help pull a lot of contaminants out of the food.

No Excuses!

With the Internet at hand and a huge number of resources available to you, there are no excuses! You eat three to five times a day. If you do it well, these sittings will help you heal. If you do it badly, the foods may well push you further into ill health. People who make excuses such as "I don't have time" or "I can't cook" are the very same people who remain plagued by nagging health complaints all their lives. So please, make the effort to improve your eating habits so that the stomach cleanse has a chance to work for you.

If you do feel a little overwhelmed by the recommendations provided here, do check out the information on pages 199-201. The *Health Freedom Secrets* online programme was designed to specifically walk you through all the dietary changes on a week-by-week basis using audio recordings, presentations and a wealth of resources. The programme enables you to implement all the information in this book – and a lot more – in a systematic and stress-free manner. Once again, details are given on pages 199-201.

Healthy, Gluten-Free Recipes

I prefer simple recipes and plain food where possible. However I hope you enjoy these specific healthy recipes – they are gluten & cow's milk free. These recipes can all be cooked in bulk, stored and re-used the following day.

Creamy Ham and Bean Stew

Ingredients:

- 1 tbsp of coconut oil
- 1 onion chopped
- 3 cloves of garlic, crushed
- 450g of gammon steaks, diced
- 1 courgette, sliced
- 1 red pepper, chopped
- 300 ml of chicken stock
- 420g of cannellini beans
- 420g of butter beans
- Black pepper
- 2 tbsp of chopped parsley
- 2 tbsp of goat's yoghurt

Instructions:

- Heat coconut oil in a large pan, add onion and garlic and cook for a few minutes until onion has softened
- Add gammon, courgette and red pepper. Fry for a few minutes until courgette starts to brown.
- Pour in chicken stock and bring to the boil. Turn down heat and simmer for 10 minutes until gammon is cooked through.
- Stir in the cannellini and butter beans, then the mustard and season with salt and pepper
- Remove from hear and stir in goat's yoghurt and parsley

Moroccan Chicken Stew with Saffron and Apricot

Ingredients:

- 10g coconut oil
- 2 onions, chopped
- 4 garlic cloves, crushed
- pinch of saffron threads
- 1 tbsp of turmeric
- 1.5 tsp of ground cumin
- 1.5 tsp of ground coriander
- 1.5 tsp of paprika
- 1 tsp of black pepper
- 1/4 of tsp of cayenne
  (avoid adding if spices irritate your stomach)
- 8 chicken thighs
- Juice of 1 lemon
- 250 ml of chicken stock
- 125g of dried apricots
- 400g of chickpeas, drained

Instructions:

- Heat oil in pan over medium heat.

- Add onion, garlic, saffron, turmeric, cumin, coriander, paprika, pepper and cayenne and cook for about 10 min or until onions are very soft.

- Add chicken, lemon juice, stock, apricots and chickpeas and bring to a simmering point. Cook gently until chicken is cooked right through.

- Serve with rice.

Pea and Ham Soup

Ingredients:

- 500g of yellow or green split peas
- 1.5 tbsp of coconut oil
- 2 onions, chopped
- 1 carrot, sliced
- 3 sticks of celery
- 1 kg of ham bones or smoked hock, chopped
- 1 bay leaf
- 2 sprigs of fresh thyme
- lemon juice to taste

Instructions:

- Place the peas in a large bowl, cover with cold water and soak for 6 hours. Drain well.

- Heat the oil in a large pan, add onion, carrot and celery and cook over low heat for 6-7 minutes.

- Add split peas, ham bones, bay leaf, thyme and 2.5 litres cold water and bring to the boil.

- Reduce heat and simmer, stir occasionally, for 2 hours. Discard the bay leaf and thyme.

- Remove the ham bones from the soup. Strip the ham from the bones and chop the meat.

- Return the meat to the soup

- Season with ground pepper and lemon juice to taste

Kale, Chorizo and Potato Soup

Ingredients:

- 225g of kale, stems removed
- 225g of chorizo sausage
  (ensure the chorizo is gluten-free)
- 675g of red potatoes
- 1.75 litres of vegetable stock
- 1 tsp of black pepper
- pinch of cayenne pepper

Instructions:

- Chop the kale finely.

- Prick sausages and place in a pan with enough water to cover. Simmer for 15 minutes. Drain and cut into thin slices.

- Cook potatoes in slightly salted water until tender (15mins). Drain and then mash, adding a little water to create a thick paste.

- Bring the vegetable stock to a boil and add the kale. Add the chorizo and simmer for 5 minutes.

- Add the potato and simmer for 20 minutes.

- Season with pepper.

Mexican Beef Chilli

Ingredients:

- 3 tbsp of coconut oil
- 350g of rump steak, cut into small pieces
- 2 onions, chopped
- 2 garlic cloves, crushed
- 2 green chillies, seeded and finely chopped
  (omit if the chilli irritates your stomach)
- 2 tbsp of mild chilli powder
  (omit if the chilli irritates your stomach)
- 1 tsp of ground cumin
- 2 bay leaves
- 2 tbsp of tomato puree
- 900ml of beef stock
- 800g of canned mixed beans
- 3 tbsp of fresh coriander
- salt and ground black pepper

Instructions:

- Heat oil in large pan and cook meat over a high heat until golden.
- Remove meat from pan.
- Reduce heat and add onions, garlic, chillies until softened.
- Add chilli powder, ground cumin and cook for 2 minutes.
- Return the meat to the pan and add bay leaves, tomato puree and beef stock. Bring to a boil
- Reduce the heat and cover the pan. Let simmer for about 45mins.
- Mash up a quarter of the beans with potato masher. Stir this into the soup.
- Add the remaining beans into soup and let simmer for 5mins.
- Season and stir in coriander.

Irish Country Soup

Ingredients:

- 15ml of coconut oil
- 650g of boneless lamb chops cut up into small pieces
- 2 small onions, quartered
- 2 leeks, thickly sliced
- 1 litre of water
- 2 large potatoes, cut into chunks
- 2 carrots, thickly sliced
- sprig of fresh thyme
- 2tbsp of chopped fresh parsley
- black pepper to taste

Instructions:

- Heat oil in large frying pan on moderate heat. Fry the lamb in batches until all of it is browned all over. Take lamb out of pan.
- Add onions to the pan and cook until softened and browned.
- Return the meat to the pan and add the leaks. Pour in the water and bring to a boil.
- Reduce heat, cover and let simmer for 1 hour.
- Add potatoes, carrots and fresh thyme and cook for 40 minutes until lamb is tender.
- Remove from the heat and let stand for 5 minutes. Skim off the fat.
- Stir in fresh parsley and serve.

Indian Lamb Soup with Rice and Coconut

Ingredients:

- 2 onions, chopped
- 6 garlic cloves, crushed
- 5cm of root ginger, grated
- 6 tbsp of olive oil
- 2 tbsp of black poppy seeds
- 1sp of cumin seeds
- 0.5 tsp of ground turmeric
- 450g of boneless lamb chops, cut into small pieces
- Quarter tsp of cayenne pepper (omit if the chilli irritates your stomach)
- 25g of rice
- 2 pints of lamb or chicken stock
- 30 ml of lemon juice
- 4 tbsp of coconut milk
- salt and pepper to taste
- fresh coriander

Instructions:

- Process onions, garlic, ginger and tbsp of olive oil in a food processor and form a paste. Set this aside.
- Use a small frying pan to heat the poppy, cumin and coriander seeds and toast for a few seconds, shaking the pan.
- Grind the seeds with a pestle and mortar. Stir in the ground turmeric.
- Heat the rest of the oil in a pan and fry the lamb in batches over a high heat until all of the pieces are browned over. Remove the lamb and set aside.

- Add onion, garlic and ginger paste to the pan and cook for 1-2 minutes, stirring continuously.

- Stir in ground spices and cook for 1 minute. Return the meat. Add the cayenne and seasoning.

- Add the beef stock and bring to the boil. Cover and simmer for 30-35 minutes.

- Stir in the rice and cover and let cook for 15 minutes.

- Add lemon juice and coconut milk for 2 minutes.

- Serve in bowls.

Spanish Fish Soup with Orange

Ingredients

- 1kg of hake fillet and the trimmings - ask the fish merchant for this.
- 2 pints of water
- 4 sweet oranges and 2 lemons
- 2tbsp of coconut oil
- 5 garlic cloves, unpeeled
- 1 tomato, peeled, seeded and chopped
- 4 small potatoes, cut into chunks
- 1 tsp of paprika
- salt and ground pepper
- 1-2 tbsp of freshly chopped parsley

Instructions:

- Cut the fillets of fish into small pieces
- Lightly salt the fillets of fish and leave on a plate
- Put the trimmings in a pan, add the water and a spiral of orange peel. Bring to a simmer, skim, then cover and cook gently for 30mins.
- Heat the oil in a large, deep pan over a high heat. Crush the garlic cloves and fry until well coloured. Discard the garlic and turn down the heat.
- Fry the onion gently until softened, adding the tomato half way through.
- Strain the hot fish stock (trimmings and water) and bring back to a boil.
- Add the potatoes and cook them for about 5mins.
- Add the fish to the soup. Cook for about 15mins. Add the squeezed orange juice and lemon juice.
- Season to taste.
- Serve in bowls

Chicken and Coconut Soup

Ingredients:

- 40g of butter or 3tbsp of coconut oil
- 1 onion, finely chopped
- 1 cup mushrooms
- 2 garlic cloves, chopped
- 2.5cm of fresh root ginger, finely chopped
- 0.5 tsp of turmeric
- 400 ml of coconut milk
- 475ml of chicken stock
- 2 lime leaves, shredded
- 1 lemon grass stalk, finely chopped
- 8 chicken thighs
- 350g of spinach, roughly chopped
- 10ml of fish sauce
- 2tbsp of freshly squeezed lime juice
- 2 shallots, thinly sliced
- 30ml of coconut oil
- salt and ground pepper

Instructions:

- Heat oil in pan. Add onion, garlic and ginger. Cook 4-5 minutes until soft.

- Stir in curry paste and turmeric and cook for a further 2-3 minutes, stirring continuously.

- Poor in two thirds of the coconut milk, cook for 5 minutes. Add the stock, lime leaves, lemon grass and chicken.

- Heat until simmering and cook for 15 minutes.

- Remove the chicken thighs

- Add the spinach to the pan and cook for a few minutes.

- Stir in the remaining coconut milk and seasoning, then process the soup in a food processor until almost smooth.

- Cut the chicken off the bones and into small pieces. Stir these into the soup with the fish sauce and lime juice.

- Reheat the soup gently until hot but do not let boil. Meanwhile stir fry the shallots separately until golden brown and then stir into the soup.

- Serve in bowls.

Smoked Mackerel and Tomato Soup

Ingredients:

- 200g of smoked mackerel fillets
- 4 tomatoes
- 1 litre of vegetable stock
- 1 lemon grass stalk, finely chopped
- 5cm of fresh galangal, finely chopped
- 4 shallots, finely chopped
- 2 garlic cloves, finely chopped
- 0.5 tsp of dried chilli flakes (omit if the chilli irritates your stomach)
- 1 tbsp of Thai fish sauce
- 3 tbsp thick tamarind juice, made by mixing tamarind paste with water
- Small bunch of fresh chives
- ½ tsp of brown sugar

Instructions:

- Chop the mackerel fillets into pieces and remove any stray bones

- Cut and deseed the tomatoes

- Pour the stock into a large pan and add the lemon grass, galangal, shallots and garlic. Bring to a boil, reduce the heat and simmer for 15mins.

- Add the fish, tomatoes, chilli flake, fish sauce, brown sugar and tamarind juice. Simmer until heated through.

- Serve in bowls.

Thai Prawn and Squash Soup

Ingredients:

- 1 butternut squash
- 1 litre of vegetable stock
- 90g of green beans
- 15ml of Thai fish sauce
- Small bunch of fresh basil
- Cooked rice to serve
- 1tsp of chilli paste (omit or reduce if the chilli irritates your stomach)

Instructions:

- Peel the butternut squash and cut in half. Scoop out the seeds with a teaspoon and discard the seeds. Then cut the squash into cubes.

- Heat the stock in a pan and add the chilli paste. Add the squash and beans. Bring to the boil and cook for 15 minutes.

- Add the fish sauce, prawns and basil. Bring to a simmering point and simmer for 3 minutes.

- Serve in bowls with the rice.

As I mentioned previously, although I know my way around the kitchen, I am not a chef. As such, I acknowledge that the above recipes may not cater for all tastes. The reason I included them is that they're all easy to make in large batches. Make sure that you do not add too many spices if your digestive system is irritated by them. We have many more recipes inside The *H Pylori Digest-Ease Recipe & Cookbook*. I think it makes the job of eating a healthy, gluten-free diet much easier and I think you'll love it!

Supermarket Foods that may Inhibit *H Pylori*

I have read many studies regarding foods that may "kill" *H pylori*. Whilst I certainly believe that chemicals in these foods can have an antibiotic effect, I am not completely convinced that, on their own, they are powerful enough to eradicate the infection. If you read a study, or some information on the Internet, stating that a food inhibits *H pylori* this does not necessarily mean that the food is capable of eradicating it. The two words *inhibit* and *eradicate* have completely different meanings.

An additional problem when reading studies is that many of them report the effects of foods *in vitro*. *In vitro* means "outside the body" and studies conducted in this manner usually involve growing *H pylori* in cultures and then exposing them to a certain food or herb to see if that substance has any effect on the bacteria. Even if the food or herb inhibits or kills the bacteria *in vitro*, there is no guarantee that the same effect will occur inside the stomach or intestine. Unfortunately many companies are looking to make a fast profit by promoting foods and products that have not been shown to exert a positive effect inside the body, or *in vivo*.

A third problem is that although certain foods have been shown to inhibit or kill *H pylori* both *in vitro* and *in vivo*, we still do not know how much of each food needs to be eaten, how often it needs to be eaten, or for how long we need to eat it! Nevertheless, as you read through the following pages you will learn that these foods can be incorporated in your programme in a number of different ways.

Based on extensive research, I have compiled a list of foods that have been shown to either inhibit or kill *H pylori in vitro*. Although these foods may not necessarily eradicate *H pylori*, incorporating them into your diet may be of benefit.

✓ **Berries (bilberry, blueberry, elderberry, raspberry, strawberry)**

✓ **Cranberry**

✓ **Broccoli**

✓ **Garlic**

✓ **Olive oil**

✓ **Tomato**

✓ **Chilli**

✓ **Ginger**

✓ **Turmeric**

Let's take a look at some of these potentially beneficial antimicrobial foods in detail. A detailed reference list can be found at **www.H-Pylori-Symptoms.com/h-pylori-studies**

Cranberries

Cranberries may help to inhibit the growth of *H pylori*. A 2008 study on a group of 271 children with *H pylori* showed very interesting results. Children who consumed cranberry juice showed an eradication rate of 16.9%, versus an eradication rate of only 1.5% in the control group.

In 2007, a group of researchers in Israel reported that cranberry juice may enhance the ability of antibiotics to clear *H pylori* from infected patients. Results from the trial involving 177 patients with *H pylori* infection, published in the journal *Molecular Nutrition & Food Research*, suggested that drinking cranberry juice during and after a weeklong antibiotic course enhanced the eradication of the bacteria by about 10 per cent.

Broccoli & Broccoli Sprouts

Broccoli contains a compound known as sulforaphane. Broccoli sprouts are known to contain the highest amount of sulforaphane. In 2002, Dr. Jed Fahey and his team of scientists showed that sulforaphane inhibited *H pylori* growth in mice .

It should be noted that other cruciferous vegetables such as cabbage, cauliflower and brussels sprouts also contain sulforaphane and may also inhibit *H pylori*. Indeed, 'vitamin U - which is not actually a vitamin at all - found in cabbage and cabbage juice is know for its ulcer-healing properties.

Olive oil

Olive oil can be used as the base for salad dressings but I recommend against cooking with it too much because it is not very stable at high temperatures. If you do want to add it to sauces, add it at the end of your meal preparation once the food has started to cool down. In other words, do not expose olive oil to high temperatures for long periods of time.

A recent study conducted by researchers from the Spanish Institute de la Grasa showed that chemicals called polyphenols contained within olive oil exhibited antibacterial activity against eight strains of *H pylori*. Three of the *H pylori* strains were said to be resistant to antibiotic treatment. Olive oil is a health promoting oil so, irrespective of whether it does kill *H pylori in vivo*, it is still good to consume it on a regular basis.

Garlic

Garlic contains allicin, which has strong antibacterial properties. Juicing one half of a fresh clove of garlic with vegetable or fruit juice consumed with a meal, or even eaten raw on its own, may help to kill unwanted organisms in your digestive tract. Be careful with garlic because too much can certainly cause unwanted bad breath and body odour as well as having the potential to irritate your digestive lining. One clove per day ought to be enough. Please avoid using a lot of garlic if you are taking blood thinning medications.

Although garlic has been shown to exhibit antimicrobial properties, its use against *H pylori* remains controversial. Some studies have failed to reveal beneficial effects on *H pylori* in people who have taken garlic in an attempt to clear the infection.

Green Tea

A recent study showed that certain components in green tea have been shown to inhibit *H pylori* and *H felis in vitro*. The green tea also helped to reduce the development of inflammation in the stomach of mice. As with other foods, the study did not indicate that green tea can eradicate *H pylori*.

Cayenne Pepper

Cayenne does not specifically work against *H pylori*, but it is believed to increase the levels of secretory IgA (sIgA) in the mucosal lining of the digestive tract. SIgA is your first line of immune defence against organisms such as *H pylori*, parasites and yeasts but its levels drop in the presence of gluten sensitivity, digestive infections and stress.

Cayenne may help to increase sIgA levels, probably by increasing blood flow to gastric mucosa. It may therefore improve the first line immune response in your stomach and intestines. You can add quarter or half a teaspoon of cayenne to a juice mix or to water. However, please be careful not to add too much cayenne as the spice may cause discomfort.

How To Control Your Blood Sugar Levels

This is such an important topic that I have designed a complete lesson in the Health Freedom Secrets programme so that you can address the issue more comprehensively.

To claim your <u>free</u> lessons and 50% Discount Coupon see pages 199-202.

Because *H pylori* infections and gluten sensitivity inhibit proper digestion and absorption of food, optimal blood sugar regulation may become a problem for you. Unstable blood sugar and the resulting stress hormone imbalances that accompany sharp blood sugar fluctuations can reduce the function of your immune system.

If your blood sugar drops too low your adrenal glands have to make more cortisol. The cortisol tells your liver to release sugar from its storage warehouses. Constant reliance on cortisol to bring the blood sugar up leads to chronically elevated cortisol levels and a weakened immune response. This all sounds rather complex, but it's quite easy to ensure that your blood sugar levels remain stable. The following recommendations will help you ensure that your blood sugar handling is optimised:

1. Try to eat every 2-3 hours. If you leave longer gaps between meals and snacks, your blood sugar may drop too low.

2. Ensure that you eat protein and fat at each meal and snack. If you only eat carbohydrates – i.e. grains, fruits & vegetables – your blood sugar may go up too quickly. It will then tend to drop too low, resulting in a rollercoaster ride that stresses your body, raising insulin and cortisol levels and inhibiting your immune system.

   Protein and fat slow down the absorption of sugar from your intestine and prevent the blood sugar rollercoaster ride. You should always eat some protein and fat before eating fruit, grains such as rice or drinking vegetable or fruit juice.

3. By avoiding gluten-containing foods, sugar and alcohol you are automatically taking a huge step towards balancing your blood sugar, hormones and immune system. These foods tend to have high sugar loads that upset the delicate balance.

How to Optimise Your Digestion

Are You Sitting Comfortably?

The sight and smell of food - or even thinking about it - triggers the release of digestive juices in your mouth and stomach. These digestive juices contain chemicals that help to break down different substances in your food and release minerals and vitamins so that they can be absorbed into your body.

Your digestive system works best when you are relaxed. One of the main problems I find is that people tend to eat on the run because of the busy and fast-paced lifestyles that they lead. It is very hard to optimise the digestive process under these circumstances.

Stress & Digestion

When your body is under stress of any kind, blood is diverted away from the digestive system and into the central nervous system and muscles. This is a survival mechanism – the so-called 'Fight or Flight' response - that is designed to help animals survive in times of stress.

If you think of a time when you were under a lot of stress, for example, after a relationship break-up or bereavement, you may recall that your appetite disappeared for a few days, or even weeks. When your body is in an emergency situation, the last thing it wants you to do is sit down and eat!

Your digestive system gradually becomes less and less efficient under stress, which is why it is so important to minimise the intake of all foods that cause stress on your body. As mentioned previously, these foods are:

- Gluten-containing foods
- Processed milk products

- Sugar
- Caffeine
- Alcohol
- Margarine and vegetable oils
- Soy
- Processed foods

As long as these foods are causing stress on your body, by producing inflammation, damaging your gut lining, lowering immune function and raising cortisol levels, I guarantee that your progress towards optimal health will be significantly slower.

Chew Your Food Properly

The digestive process begins when you chew your food. Chewing breaks down solid food and mixes it with saliva. By chewing food adequately, you increase the surface area of the mixture so that acid and enzymes can break down the food more effectively in the stomach.

Saliva also contains amylase, an enzyme that helps to break down the carbohydrates found in fruit, vegetables and beans. If you do not chew your food thoroughly, you effectively skip the first stage of digestion, which places greater pressure on your stomach and makes the entire digestive process less efficient.

Chewing thoroughly also helps to release parasites that may be hidden in your food. The acid in your stomach will be more effective in killing the parasites once they are exposed. If they remain hidden in large chunks or particles of food, the stomach juices may not have adequate contact with the parasites to kill them. You should aim to chew your food until it is liquid. Chewing anywhere from 20-40 times per mouthful should accomplish this.

How to Eat More Raw Foods by Using Vegetable Juicing

Juicing fresh vegetables and fruits is a fantastic way to accelerate your journey towards optimal health. There are three main reasons why juicing will help you:

1. **Juicing helps you absorb more nutrients from vegetables.** If you have *H pylori*, gluten sensitivity and associated gastrointestinal damage, you may not be digesting your food effectively. Even if you are eating fresh, organic foods, you may not be deriving optimal benefit from them because you simply cannot break them down. Juicing essentially pre-digests your vegetables thereby reducing stress on your digestive system and allowing you to derive optimum benefit from the vegetables.

2. **Juicing enables you to eat raw vegetables easily.** The cooking process actually removes nutrients from many vegetables. Through juicing, you have easy access to all the nutrients in the raw vegetables without the need to expend energy digesting them.

3. **You can add a wider variety of vegetables to your diet**. If you do not rotate your food regularly, you run the risk of developing food allergies to the foods you eat most. This is especially the case if you have a damaged digestive system. Juicing allows you to rotate your vegetables and also eat ones that you may not like because you can mix them with other vegetables and foods.

Vegetable Juice versus Fruit Juice

Fruit juices generally contain more sugar than vegetable juices. Major fluctuations in blood sugar levels are a significant cause of stress on your body and should be avoided. Along with mental and emotional stress, hidden inflammation from gluten and digestive infections, unstable blood sugar can place a huge demand on your adrenal glands and other stress-coping mechanisms.

You should therefore only juice small amounts of fruit and take care with vegetables such as carrots and beets. These below-ground vegetables are higher in sugar and can cause blood sugars to rise too steeply, leading to a sharp drop.

Nevertheless, one or two small carrots and a small amount of beet can work well to enhance flavour and add additional nutrients to your juice, as can green apples and pears. It is also worth noting that the less ripe fruits are, the less sugar they will contain, but the harder they will be to digest.

Juicing For Breakfast

Breakfast is typically a meal where people do not eat vegetables. However it is easy to consume vegetables for breakfast if you juice them. Some of the best vegetables to juice are:

✓ Celery

✓ Cucumber

✓ Courgette / Zucchini

✓ Fennel

✓ Carrot

✓ Beets

✓ Apple

✓ Pear

Do not use more than one to two small carrots or a small piece of beet per sitting. If you would like to add a little fruit, I suggest half of or one small peeled apple/pear but no more than that otherwise your blood sugar may go too high.

The next set of vegetables to introduce can include:

✓ Lettuce (all kinds)

✓ Endive

✓ Escarole

✓ Spinach (baby spinach is good)

✓ Cabbage

✓ Bok Choy

✓ Asparagus

Finally, you can introduce the bitter leafy vegetables to taste. These tend to be a little harder to digest. If you feel digestive symptoms after drinking vegetable juice make a note of the vegetables you have used. You may find a pattern where, for example, every time you drink some cabbage juice, you get stomach pain or wind.

✓ Kale

✓ Collard Greens (with leaves attached to stalks for optimal nutrition)

It is not essential to add all these different vegetables – use the ones that taste pleasant to you and experiment with them to find the combinations that you like most. If you experience any increases in your symptoms when you add some of the green leafy vegetables, particularly bloating, stomach pain or cramp, it's probably best to leave those vegetables out – not everyone can deal with large quantities of raw vegetables.

Juicing As Part of a Meal

I prefer to drink my vegetable juice 15 minutes after a meal. This ensures that the juice mixes with the protein and fat of the meal and doesn't cause blood sugar fluctuations. I eat the bulk of my meal first and then have the juice right at the end.

This is an excellent way to achieve a balanced meal with lots of high quality nutrition and it makes it easier to consume vitamins and minerals at breakfast.

Juicing As a Snack

I do not recommend using vegetable juice as a snack without adding protein and fat. If you would like to take vegetable juice as part of a snack, make sure you have it after some protein and fat: a boiled egg or some roast chicken or beef slices, for example.

Making Juice Itself into a Balanced Meal or Snack

Vegetable juice is packed full of valuable vitamins and minerals but it does not contain fat or protein. For this reason, in its own right it should not be used as a meal. You can, however, add other foods to the juice to make it into a more balanced meal. Some of the following recommendations may not be to your taste but they are worth trying if you're feeling adventurous. Have fun playing around with the recipes and see which ones suit your particular taste. You will need a blender to make these recipes.

- Use a raw egg. This will provide great fats and protein to the juice. Only use organic eggs, however, as the battery-farmed eggs may contain harmful bacteria, including *H pylori*! It is not recommended to add raw eggs into the juice if you are pregnant because there is a possibility that raw eggs can lead to biotin deficiency.

- Add a tablespoon of organic, cold pressed extra virgin olive oil. This will add plenty of healthy fat to your juice and may help inhibit *H pylori* growth.

- Add coconut juices from a fresh coconut, or bits of shredded coconut for texture. Coconut is a healthy source of fats and oils and its lauric acid content is known to have antibiotic properties that may be helpful in controlling *H pylori*.

- Fresh or frozen cranberries may be blended into your juice. Cranberries are packed full of important antioxidant nutrients and have been shown to inhibit the growth of *H pylori*.

- Ginger adds a lovely kick to the juice and is also great for digestive health. A small piece of stem or root ginger works well. Add to taste.

- A single clove of raw garlic can be very useful as a weapon against *H pylori*. I don't recommend using more than one clove though as the juice may become too strong and cause a burning sensation in your throat and stomach. Add to taste.

- Consider adding a protein powder to your juice, or add your vegetable juice to a smoothie recipe. The quality of the protein powder is important and I do not recommend using brands other than those listed on the smoothie recipe page at **www.H-Pylori-Symptoms.com/smoothies**.

Smoothies can also be used to help provide healing nutrients for the stomach and intestinal lining. Amino acids such as glutamine can assist greatly in repairing damaged gut lining caused by the likes of gluten and digestive infections.

> **My Favourite Juice Recipes – always taken at the end of a meal and I only take 4-6oz in one sitting:**
>
> 1. *2 x small carrots, 1-2 sticks celery, 5-6 large handfuls baby spinach, small cut of ginger stem (I sometimes add ½ a small apple instead of carrot)*
>
> 2. *2 x small carrots, ½ cucumber or courgette/zucchini, 3-4 large handfuls of spinach, small cut of fresh ginger stem.*
>
> 3. *1 x small green apple, 1 x carrot, ½ cucumber and a little ginger root.*

I always juice the garlic and ginger first and finish with the carrot or celery because there is a lot more juice in the latter. This helps to push through the juice from the other vegetables through the machine. Please note that, according to research, the best active ingredients to include in juices or smoothies for working against *H pylori* are as follows, but I repeat that I do not think these foods alone are potent enough to completely clear *H pylori* in most people:

✓ Garlic

✓ Olive Oil

✓ Coconut

✓ Cranberries

✓ Raspberries

✓ Strawberries

✓ Blueberries

✓ Ginger

Always ensure that you drink your juice as soon as you have made it. If you leave it standing, the juice will oxidise. To see an example of this just juice a carrot and see it turn from orange to brown in only a few minutes, or cut an apple in half and watch the flesh quickly turn brown.

Water & Hydration Guidelines

"Water and Hydration" is the first topic we cover in the *Health Freedom Secrets* programme, and for good reason. Depending on which book you read and how hydrated you are, your body is said to be comprised of 60-70% water. Water is absolutely vital for:

✓ Keeping your skin healthy

✓ Maintaining your body temperature

✓ Digestion, nutrient absorption and elimination of food

✓ Lubrication and cushioning of joints and in your spine

✓ Removing toxic chemicals from your body

✓ Creating energy inside your cells to drive metabolism

Without water, you simply cannot exist! If you do not consume enough pure water, or you drink caffeine-laden sodas, coffee, black tea, red bull or other sports drinks, your body may well become dehydrated because caffeine is a diuretic.

As you become more and more dehydrated your body actually pulls water out of certain areas and into your central nervous system, where it is needed most. Your brain and central nervous system are the most important areas of your body in terms of survival, so they have priority over water distribution at the expense of areas such as the digestive system, skin and joints.

Doctor F. Batmanghelidj tells us in his book *Your Body's Many Cries for Water* that dehydration of only 1% can lead to psychological disorders such as 'brain fog' and depression. If you're dehydrated to a greater extent, many other physiological adaptations are made by your body. In your mind, picture bare earth that hasn't seen rain for many weeks. It's parched and full of cracks. Well, if you don't stay hydrated and you have *H pylori*, your stomach could end up looking like that bare earth. Your body will pull water from the mucous linings of your stomach in order to satisfy the needs of the central nervous system.

If you have *H pylori*, this is disastrous because the water in your mucous membranes helps to protect against the acidity of your stomach. When your mucosal lining is damaged through lack of hydration and *H pylori*, acid gets into those damaged areas. This is akin to pouring vinegar into a cut on your finger!

Over time the effect of the acid on unprotected mucous membranes can lead to gastric and duodenal ulcers. Dr. Batmanghelidj was able to cure more than 10,000 cases of ulcer disease during his time in a prisoner of war camp, using only water. I highly recommend that you read his book.

Water is also vital for enzyme function in your digestive system. Remember that if you have *H pylori* your digestion will already be adversely affected because the inflammation caused by the *H pylori* damages cells in your stomach that are responsible for acid and enzyme production. Without adequate water, whatever enzymes are left in your stomach will not function properly and you will not be able to digest your food. If you are unable to digest food you may not be able to absorb nutrients like B-vitamins, vitamins A, D, E & K, magnesium, calcium and iron.

Back pain can also be caused or aggravated by dehydration because your body will pull water out of the spinal discs. This causes compression in the discs and can result in back and neck pain. Back pain is common in people who have compromised digestion and can be a symptom of *H pylori*.

If you are struggling with weight gain you may find that it is partly the result of dehydration. Water helps your body to eliminate toxins. If you are dehydrated, this detoxification operation will not work efficiently. Until you are hydrated and body is able to detoxify the chemicals, the fat will not be released. In this case, being dehydrated is a bit like trying to clean your kitchen without having access to a wet cloth.

How Much Water Should You Drink?

I've no doubt that you've read or been told to drink 8 x 8oz glasses of water per day. This is a reasonable starting point but the trouble is that a 50kg woman will need a lot less water than a 120kg man. Seasonal differences in temperature and the amount of exercise or physical activity you do will also affect your water requirements.

Using the colour of your urine can be a good way of assessing your hydration levels. If you are well hydrated your urine should be very light or pale yellow. If your urine is a dark yellow / orange colour, it may indicate that you are dehydrated. Note that if you are taking a supplement that contains vitamin B_2 (riboflavin), your urine may turn bright yellow/green in colour.

As a rough guide, try to drink an ounce of water per pound of bodyweight, each day. For example, if you weigh 100lbs, drink 50oz water; if you are 250lbs, aim to drink 125oz water.

Is Tap Water Good For You?

Pure, clean water is the best option for quenching your thirst and supporting your body. Unfortunately, in our modern world, tap-water is not as clean as you may think. I have not used tap water for a long time and I can now actually smell the chlorine in it from a couple of feet away, especially if it's a full bathtub's worth!

In *The Healthy Water Report* Dr. Martin Fox states that:

"Over 2100 organic and inorganic drinking water contaminants have been identified in the U.S. drinking water supply since 1974. Out of these 2100, 190 of the contaminants have confirmed adverse health effects."

Tap water has chlorine added to it to kill potentially harmful bugs. The problem is that the chlorine may also wipe out the good bacteria in your digestive system and this is completely counter-productive if you are trying to heal gut infections such as *H pylori*.

Fluorine is also added to tap water in many areas with the premise that it is good for your teeth. However data from the World Health Organisation shows that there is absolutely no difference in tooth decay rates in countries that use fluoridated water compared to those that do not. In 2007, the American Dental Association actually advised dentists not to give fluoride to babies because of its adverse effects on bone growth.

In addition to chlorine and fluoride, consider that traces of these other potentially damaging chemicals are regularly found in tap water:

- Pesticides
- Mercury

- Arsenic

- Aluminium

- Residues of pharmaceutical products (birth control pills, antidepressants, painkillers, shampoos plus many other chemical compounds).

The problem with these chemicals is that many of them are tasteless, colourless and odourless, which means that you have no way of knowing they're in your water. However even in tiny concentrations they can still do a lot of harm over a period of many years.

Sodas & Fruit Juices

Sodas and fruit juices are loaded with sugar and the former often contain sugar or, in the diet varieties, artificial sweeteners. It's very important to minimise both. Be wary of so-called 'healthy fruit juices'. Unless the juice is being prepared in front of you from fresh fruit, or you are preparing it yourself, stay away as the juices are processed and contain little nutritional value other than sugar.

If you are drinking organically grown vegetable juices you will also be getting a healthy source of water. Celery, carrot and cucumber are particularly useful for helping with hydration.

Where Should You Get Your Water?

I used to drink and recommend bottled water. However plastic bottles can leach chemicals into the water while they are on the shelves and may also contain the potentially toxic metal antimony. They are also devastating to the environment and use a great deal of oil in their manufacture.

Water bottled in glass can be excellent – Evian, for example – although it tends to be quite expensive. However I learned a nice trick to cut costs if you want to use this option. Go to a local shop, café or restaurant and ask for the name of their wholesale water supplier. You may be able to buy glass-bottled water in weekly, fortnightly or even monthly batches at a very inexpensive wholesale rate.

If you are able to afford one, reverse osmosis (RO) filter systems can be a great tool for purifying your water. These systems work by squeezing water through a semi-permeable membrane that is tiny enough to keep out contaminants while letting only pure water through. RO systems are often used to convert seawater into drinking water.

You can buy three different types of system:

1.   A counter-top RO system.

2.   An under the sink system.

3.   A whole-house filtration system.

If these systems are out of your price range, some filtration is better than none and a standard table-top water filter will certainly be beneficial over drinking water straight from your tap.

To get <u>free</u> access to the Water & Hydration lesson from the Health Freedom Secrets programme see pages 199-202.

Phase Three – The Stomach Cleanse

The *stomach cleanse* protocol is the part of your programme where you use nutritional supplements that have been scientifically and clinically shown to exert an anti-*H pylori* effect. Because I am not a licensed medical professional, I am obliged to recommend that you seek your doctor's approval before beginning the stomach cleanse.

When I had *H pylori*, my primary symptoms were severe heartburn, stomach pain, morning nausea, belching and constipation. All these symptoms improved within three days of beginning the stomach cleanse I'm about to teach you and were completely gone within 4 weeks. I am not claiming that each one of you will experience the same rate of recovery, but the programme works extremely well for the majority of people.

The beauty of the stomach cleanse is that it can be used on its own, or alongside triple therapy antibiotics (or quadruple and sequential therapies, should your doctor be in a position to prescribe them for you). The stomach cleanse can be used, before, after or alongside antibiotic therapy, which makes it completely compatible with medical treatments, not opposed to them.

It is my personal belief that nutritionists, functional medicine practitioners and other naturally orientated practitioners should look to work alongside medical practitioners. We have an unfortunate situation whereby physicians and natural practitioners are at loggerheads with one another, each claiming the other's approach doesn't work!

There is a time and place for all therapies. Some people respond well to medical treatment when others don't. The same is true for natural therapies as well. Nobody can claim that his or her approach works *every* time and with every person and I am no different. Herbal protocols and diet changes won't keep me alive if I'm hit by a bus, so while I prefer to promote a natural approach, be aware that I also write plenty of letters to doctors recommending that they prescribe antibiotics for patients! I have an exceptional success rate with my clients, but on the odd occasion I see a case that proves to be extremely difficult to resolve, even with medical support. This is usually because a lot of 'collateral damage' has been caused by long-term food intolerances, infections and other physiological imbalances.

Timing of the Stomach Cleanse

I highly recommend that you only run a stomach cleanse protocol after you have followed the *H Pylori Diet* programme for *8-12 weeks, or 60-90 days*. The 8-12 week nutrition programme will ensure that inflammation in your digestive system has had a chance to heal somewhat. However if your symptoms are debilitating or you are not experiencing relief from using only the nutrition programme, you can begin running the stomach cleanse sooner or even straight away.

Remember that the *H Pylori Diet* on its own probably won't be enough to eradicate your *H pylori*. The purpose of adjusting your diet is to enhance your overall health, reduce stress and inflammation and bring your hormones more into balance so that when you begin the stomach cleanse your body is stronger and more able to work synergistically with the cleanse.

If you do not follow the *H Pylori Diet* recommendations I have presented there is a chance that the supplements – and even triple therapy antibiotics - will not work for the following reasons:

1. Continuing to eat gluten, processed cow's milk and soy products may result in *zero* reduction to the inflammation in your digestive system. As a result your cortisol level may remain high, which inhibits your immune system.

2. Inflammation in your digestive system can lead to the formation of 'pockets' in the intestinal lining where

bacteria and parasites may 'hide'. The pits in your digestive lining, known as the *crypts of lieberkhun*, become enclosed by the inflamed tissue and can harbour bacteria and parasites. This phenomenon is called *crypt hyperplasia*. Because the crypts become deep and enclosed, the supplements or meds you take may not come into contact with hidden *H pylori* organisms.

3. Your immune system will be adversely affected if you eat processed, packaged foods, sugar and caffeine. These foods will not provide you with the nutrients required to be healthy.

What Are The Best Natural Herbs & Supplements For *H Pylori*?

In my experience natural programmes can be just as effective as Triple Therapy in helping you overcome the challenges caused by *H pylori*. However it is very important to understand exactly how to run the natural programme properly so that you do not waste time and money. Here are the aspects you *must* know:

1. Exactly which herbal and supplements to use to get maximum benefit.

2. Where to obtain products that contain herbs and nutrients that have the highest potency and quality.

3. The correct dosage of each supplement: if you do not use the right dose, the programme might not work.

4. Whether to take the product with or without food.

5. The duration of the programme: a programme that is too short may not work, or may only work temporarily.

Scientific research has shown that a number of natural products can inhibit and kill *H pylori*. However there are also a number of products that are promoted on the Internet and in health food shops that may not necessarily be optimal choices.

This section is designed to help you negotiate the supplement minefield so that you use the most effective products with the least financial risk. Remember that you're reading one person's opinion and I am not claiming that my way is the *only* way. However these products have been used by many highly successful doctors and practitioners around the world.

Berberine

Berberine is a constituent of herbs such as goldenseal, barberry and Oregon grape. It has been shown to have broad-spectrum antibiotic activity. Studies *in vitro* have demonstrated that berberine can inhibit *H pylori*, but it may not be potent enough to eradicate the organism.

Deglycyrrhizinated Liquorice Root (DGL)

DGL is a well established anti-ulceration and mucosal healing agent. DGL can coat and soothe the intestinal lining and promote the healing of inflamed tissue and ulcers. Research suggests that flavonoids in liquorice have impressive antimicrobial activity against *H pylori*. The flavonoids have actually been shown to have antimicrobial activity against strains of *H pylori* that were resistant to clarithromycin and amoxicillin, two of the primary antibiotics used in triple therapy. Some forms of liquorice can elevate blood pressure but because DGL has low glycyrrhizin levels it is generally safe to take if you have high blood pressure.

Manuka Honey

Manuka honey comes from New Zealand. It is often promoted as a food that can kill *H pylori*. Whilst this may be the case, it is worth remembering that honey is essentially sugar. We know that *Candida* and other species of yeast thrive on sugar and we also know that there is a close relationship between *H pylori* infection and *Candida* overgrowth. For this reason, I do not recommend the use of manuka honey for people who have digestive problems as I believe there are better alternatives.

But you should not rule out its use as it may help you on an individual basis.

Mastic Gum

The protocol I originally learned in my functional medicine training involved the use of mastic gum and a supplement called Bio-HPF, which contains several herbs as well as bismuth. Interestingly, bismuth medications are recommended as part of quadruple therapy protocols alongside antibiotics. If you use bismuth products they can turn your stool darker and it is not recommended that you use bismuth for longer than 60-days.

Despite doctors and practitioners reporting great success using the mastic and Bio-HPF programme, it didn't work for me. My symptoms actually worsened when I started taking these supplements. Despite my poor reaction to the mastic programme, there is quite a large body of research demonstrating its efficacy against *H pylori* and mastic gum has been shown to kill *H pylori in vitro.*

Matula Herbal Formula™

My preferred cleanse involves a 30-day course of Matula Herbal Formula. Matula Herbal Formula resolved my symptoms very quickly. In fact I was staggered by the speed at which my symptoms eased using the product. I have had detailed discussions with the Matula staff and they have a very open and honest approach to business.

I read the technical report on Matula that was put together by Professor Patrick J. D. Bouic of the Department of Medical Microbiology at Stellenbosch University in South Africa and whilst this is not strictly independent research, it makes for impressive reading. *In vitro* testing on *H pylori* revealed that every time Matula came into contact with *H pylori*, it killed 93% of the organisms. Although these tests were performed *in vitro* (outside the body), the level of clinical success I have observed using Matula has confirmed its effectiveness.

In my opinion, *Matula Herbal Formula* has several advantages over competing products:

- It tends to work very quickly (30-days is usually enough – supplements such as mastic gum usually need to be taken for a minimum of 60-days).

- Some practitioners advise that mastic gum should be taken for 4-6 months.

- It has a pleasant taste.

- It is very simple to implement and particularly good for people who do not enjoy taking capsules, or who are already taking supplements in capsule form and do not want to take more.

- *In vitro* studies have shown that Matula is effective in inhibiting *Candida albicans* overgrowth in addition to eradicating *H pylori*.

- The company offers a money back guarantee if the product fails to eradicate *H pylori*, as long as a stool retest confirms eradication failure.

You will doubtless read mixed reports about Matula on the Internet. Because it is a relatively expensive product, people are naturally disappointed if they do not feel better when they take it. But as I taught you in part one of this book and in the *H Pylori Diet* section, just taking a 'miracle' product, whether it's a pill, a tea or a potion, won't work if your symptoms are being caused by the food that you eat, dehydration and other infections! Unfortunately some folk still believe that they can eat McDonalds three times a day and take a product like Matula to cure all their ills. I'd like to encourage you not to believe everything you read on the Internet, particularly if people have written the material in an emotionally charged state.

Siberian Pine Nut Oil

I personally do not have any experience of using pine nut oil. I have read mixed reports about it on the Internet and have received emails from people who have used it without any success. To date I have not seen any research that proves its efficacy. Nevertheless there are some positive testimonials on some websites. Recall that olive oil has been shown to contain antimicrobial properties against *H pylori*. It is certainly possible that pine nut oil contains similar properties that help it work against the bacteria.

Sulforaphane

Sulforaphane is a naturally occurring chemical found in cruciferous vegetables such as broccoli, cabbage and brussels sprouts. A number of studies have demonstrated that it has the capacity to inhibit *H pylori*. Eating cruciferous vegetables, especially broccoli sprouts, will ensure that you get plenty of sulforaphane, but it is also available in capsule form from several supplement manufacturers, including a product called *Broccomax*.

Vitamin C

Some studies have suggested that vitamin C may inhibit and even kill *H pylori*. In a review of the literature, Dr. Alan Gaby, MD concludes that vitamin C therapy for *H pylori* may be clinically relevant, but that more research is needed to determine the optimal dosing and programme duration. Even if vitamin C does not eradicate *H pylori*, it is still worth taking a controlled dose because studies clearly show that vitamin C levels in the stomach lining can be reduced when *H pylori* is present, largely as a result of the inflammatory and oxidative stress caused by the infection. Vitamin C is also an excellent nutrient for assisting with gut healing.

'Vitamin U'

Vitamin U – also known as MSM – is found in raw cabbage. In fact, vitamin U is not actually a vitamin at all. Cabbage juice has been studied extensively in Russia and other Eastern European countries for the healing of damaged and eroded intestinal mucosa. It is not actually a vitamin *per se*. It appears to enhance the healing of damaged tissue and may assist in healing ulcers.

Zinc-L-Carnosine

To my knowledge, zinc-l-carnosine has not been shown to have antimicrobial properties against *H pylori*. However it is excellent for repairing damage to the stomach lining, and may assist in healing ulcers. It can be taken alongside any of the antimicrobial agents to augment the healing process.

Specific Products

Matula Herbal Formula™

Matula Herbal Formula is herbal tea comprised of a blend of herbs that grow in a small geographical area in the Cape Mountains of South Africa. The Matula is packaged into teabags. You simply make a cup of tea twice daily and drink it on an empty stomach. Because it is a highly specialised product, Matula must be ordered online and is not available in stores, unless the store has an agreement with the company to buy and resell the product. Unfortunately, due to AQIS restrictions, Matula is not allowed into Australia, so if you're in Australia please do pay special attention to the other products discussed below.

Gastromend-HP™

Gastromend-HP™ is an excellent product that is based on mastic gum. It is manufactured by the US company Designs for Health. Rather than simply using mastic gum in the capsules, Designs for Health have also added vitamin U, vitamin C and

DGL for their antimicrobial activity against *H pylori* and their ability to heal the stomach and intestinal lining. Gastromend-HP™ also contains zinc-l-carnosine. The inclusion of these substances means that you do not need to buy separate bottles of each product, which helps to keep the cost of your stomach cleanse down and also makes the cleanse more convenient. Gastromend HP can be ordered from the US and UK and is not restricted in countries such as Australia, where import regulations are very strict.

Bio-HPF®

Bio-HPF is an excellent supplement made by Biotics Research Corporation. It contains bismuth citrate and berberine, which may inhibit *H pylori*. The product also contains DGL and several other herbs that have been shown to support the lining of the digestive tract. Bio-HPF can be ordered from the US and UK and is not restricted in countries such as Australia, where import regulations are very strict.

BroccoMax™

Broccomax™ is a supplement from Jarrow Formulas that contains broccoli extract. You may recall that broccoli and other cruciferous vegetables contain sulforaphane, which has been shown to have antimicrobial activity against *H pylori*. This product can be purchased from the US and UK and is not restricted in countries such as Australia, where import regulations are very strict.

Which Products & When?

The stomach cleanse protocol is designed to help inhibit *H pylori*. Some of you will experience significant relief as a result of following the stomach cleanse and altering your diet according to the recommendations in this book.

1. Stomach Cleanse – uses herbs that have been scientifically proven to inhibit and/or kill *Helicobacter pylori*.

2. Yeast Cleanse – uses an herbal programme to clear yeast overgrowth.

3. Probiotic Replacement – to provide nutrients and good bacteria to help repair the structure and function of your digestive system.

As discussed above, many natural substances have been shown to have antimicrobial properties against *H pylori*. We have already explored specific foods that you can incorporate into your diet for this purpose. The problem lies in sorting these herbs and nutrients into those that only inhibit the organism and those that are actually strong enough to eradicate it.

The only real way to determine whether these herbs work in practice is to use them in a clinical setting. The protocols I have provided below have a proven track record and have been used not only by me, but by many leading doctors and natural healthcare practitioners worldwide, over many years and with thousands of patients.

My preferred protocol is Matula Herbal Formula because of its efficiency, ease of application, competitive pricing and the fact that the company offers a100% money back guarantee if follow-up stool testing indicates that it has not been effective (the company honours its guarantee, so using Matula truly is risk-free).

With your doctor's blessing, run the protocol below for the specified duration. Matula Herbal Formula alone is usually effective, but you can add the other products into your programme simultaneously if desired. Alternatively, take them once you have completed your Matula programme.

Stomach Cleanse	upon arising	with breakfast	mid morning	with lunch	mid afternoon	with dinner	before sleep
Essential							
Matula Herbal Formula™ 30-days	1 cup						1 cup
Optional / Additional							
Gastromend-HP 60-days	2						2
Bio-HPF® (optional) 60-days		2		2		2	
Broccomax™ (optional) 60-days	2						2

To complete this protocol you will need to purchase the following:

✓ 1 box of Matula Herbal Formula for 30-days.

If you would like to make your stomach cleanse protocol more comprehensive, add the following products:

✓ 2 bottles of Gastromend-HP for 30-days
  (4 bottles for 60-days).

✓ 1 bottles of Bio-HPF for 30-days (4 bottles for 60-days).

✓ 2 bottles of Broccomax for 30-days (4 bottles for
  60-days).

I appreciate that ordering all these products at once may be expensive. If you do have budget restrictions, I recommend that you first order Matula Herbal Formula and take it for 30-days. After this time it may be that you do not need to order the other products. If you want to use the programme with maximal effect, take the products together, as it is laid out above.

Remember that you can order the Matula Herbal Formula completely risk-free. If it fails to eradicate your *H pylori* the company offers a 100% money back guarantee. *Please read the company's terms and conditions carefully* for details.

How To Order The Stomach Cleanse Products

- **Matula Herbal Formula™**
  www.Perfectly-Natural-Health.com
  Order from here if you are anywhere in the world
  except Australia*

- **Gastromend-HP™**
  Australia, US & Canada: **www.MossNutrition.com**
  UK & Europe: **www.NutritionGeeks.co.uk**

- **Bio-HPF®**
  Australia, US & Canada:
  www.bioticsresearch.com/node/1637
  UK & Europe: Nutrilink Ltd 08450 760 402

- **Broccomax™** (sulforaphane)
  Australia, US & Canada: **www.iherb.com**
  UK & Europe: **www.Health-Interlink.com/products**

Important Notes for Australian Customers

Unfortunately, Matula Herbal Formula is not available in Australia due to AQIS restrictions. Customs regulations prohibit importation of the product into the country. If you are in Australia, use the other products as listed.

Possible Side Effects & Precautions

Any food, drug or herb has the potential to cause a reaction. I have received emails from people who did not react well to mastic gum and from people who are allergic to broccoli. I have seen cases where Matula caused side effect as well. However the chances of suffering side-effects from the natural products are miniscule compared with the risks associated with the use of triple therapy. Nevertheless if you do feel any side effects from the stomach cleanse protocol, here is the action to take:

- Stop taking the supplements immediately.

- See if your side effects go away.

- When all is normal again, reintroduce one supplement, at half dose.

- If all is ok, then increase to the full dose.

- If all is ok, then introduce any other supplements, one at a time, following the same process.

You may also prefer to introduce all products one-by-one in the first place, ensuring that you do not develop any reactions to the individual products. I would like to reiterate that the chances of experiencing side-effects are small but if you are unsure of how you may respond to the protocols or have any questions, please feel free to contact us at **Office@HPExperts.com**.

Can The Stomach Cleanse Be Used Alongside Triple Therapy?

The stomach cleanse can be used alongside triple therapy. It can also be used before or after the antibiotic treatment. However I do not recommend using Gastromend-HP alongside Triple Therapy because the DGL component of the product may reduce the efficacy of the antibiotics.

You Can Make Triple Therapy More Effective

Although I am an advocate of natural medicine, I do not totally refute the efficacy of triple therapy. Antibiotics and proton pump inhibitors certainly have their place in treatment protocols. Many people do have success when they use triple therapy, so please do consider your options. Research demonstrates that triple therapy may be enhanced by the use of both bovine lactoferrin and probiotics and that the addition of these supplements can reduce side-effects.

Lactoferrin

Lactoferrin is a substance that is found in mother's milk and has immune enhancing properties. Several studies have demonstrated that lactoferrin from cow's milk can enhance the eradication rate of *H pylori* when it is used alongside triple therapy. Lactoferrin can be purchased in capsule form and it is also available in certain whey protein powders. You can purchase lactoferrin at the link below:

Laktoferrin (Allergy Research Group)

Australia, Canada & US: **www.MossNutrition.com**
UK & Europe: Nutrilink Ltd 08450 760 402

Whey Cool™ (Designs for Health)

Australia, Canada & US: **www.MossNutrition.com**
UK & Europe: **www.NutritionGeeks.co.uk**

I personally consume 2 scoops Whey Cool after exercise and may also make smoothies using the protein blended with some fruit, coconut milk and a raw egg if I am rushed for time at breakfast. The whey cool tends to be tolerated very well even by folk who have lactose intolerance and milk allergy.

Probiotics

Researchers have also discovered that the use of probiotics such as *Lactobacillus* can also enhance the efficacy of triple therapy as well as reducing side effects. There are many probiotic supplements on the market but it is important to make sure you purchase high quality products. I have had great success using the following brand:

Probiotic Synergy™ (Designs for Health)

Australia, Canada & US: **www.MossNutrition.com**
UK & Europe: **www.NutritionGeeks.co.uk**

Saccharomyces boulardii

S. boulardii is a type of yeast. It is not related to *Candida albicans*. In fact, *S boulardii* has been studied extensively and has been shown to improve immune function, reduce inflammation and compete favourably against pathogens in the digestive tract. I often use it alongside probiotics to help clients enhance their digestive function after the stomach cleanse. Designs For Health do a good product called *Floramyces™* for this purpose.

General Yeast & Fungal Cleanse & Probiotics

As I taught you in part one of *The H Pylori Diet*, *H pylori* infection is strongly associated with the presence of yeast and that the treatment of *H pylori* can lead to yeast and fungal overgrowth. It can be helpful, therefore, to run a yeast and fungal cleanse and probiotic programme *after* the stomach cleanse but I would recommend that you run a comprehensive stool test to identify exactly what your individual requirements are.

How To Order The Yeast Cleanse & Probiotic Products

- *GI Microb-X™*
  Australia, US & Canada: **www.MossNutrition.com**
  UK & Europe: **www.NutritionGeeks.co.uk**

- *Oil of Oregano*
  Australia, US & Canada: **www.MossNutrition.com**
  UK & Europe: **www.NutritionGeeks.co.uk**

- *Probiotic Synergy™*
  Australia, US & Canada: **www.MossNutrition.com**
  UK & Europe: **www.NutritionGeeks.co.uk**

- *Floramyces™*

Basic Yeast/Fungal Cleanse	upon arising	with breakfast	mid morning	with lunch	mid afternoon	with dinner	before sleep
GI Microb-X™ capsules 30-days	2						2
Oil of Oregano 30-days		2				2	
Probiotics							
Probiotic Synergy™ 30 days		2				2	
Floramyces™ 30 days		2				2	

Although the yeast/fungal and probiotic phases of the programme can be very helpful, it is my personal opinion that your money is better spent on comprehensive lab testing that will enable you to pinpoint *exactly* which additional cleanses you need. For example, if you have a parasite or other bacterial infection, which is very common, you may benefit from a completely different set of products. Remember that the tests are available to you irrespective of your geographical location as we have distributors in North America, the UK and Australia.

Can Children Use The Stomach Cleanse?

I have successfully used the stomach cleanse programme to help children overcome *H pylori* related symptoms. I usually recommend that children simply take half the adult dose of the natural supplements. I also see amazing results when children follow *The H Pylori Diet*. If you have questions about your child's digestive symptoms, energy levels, attention span or skin, please contact our office by emailing **Office@HPExperts.com**.

How Do You Know *H pylori* Has Gone?

The only way of knowing whether *H pylori* bacteria have been eradicated is to run a retest. Even if your symptoms have gone, you may still carry small numbers of *H pylori* bacteria and these organisms have the potential to spread again if you do not make sure that eradication is complete. Symptoms can go away completely only to return a few weeks or months later. I am a firm believer that if you are going to run a programme to eliminate *H pylori* you might as well do it properly because it will save a lot of time, hassle and money in the long term.

What Is The Best Way of Re-Testing?

Many people make the mistake of *not retesting* after treatment. Others make the mistake of using the wrong test, or testing too soon after they have finished their triple therapy or stomach cleanse.

Here are some key points that you must follow when retesting:

- Do not use a blood test because it can remain positive for up to 3-5 years after *H pylori* has gone. Your body will continue to make antibodies against *H pylori* and this test can give a false-positive.

- Always wait *at least 4 weeks* after finishing your treatment (natural or medical) before retesting so that you obtain an accurate test result. If you take the test too soon, you risk false negative or false positive results.

- I do not recommend the use of a breath test for retesting because I have seen many cases where the breath test has been positive for *H pylori* but a stool test has revealed no *H pylori*, but instead other infections or *Candida* overgrowth. I suspect that the breath test may give false positive results when other bugs are present.

Ideally, the only test that should be used to confirm the eradication of *H pylori* is a stool test. I run a comprehensive stool panel with my clients because the test can:

- Confirm *H pylori* eradication.

- Identify whether or not *Candida* overgrowth is present.

- Identify whether you need probiotics and which ones.

- Tell you whether other parasites, yeasts and bacteria are present.

If you are having difficulty accessing the appropriate digestive testing, or the testing you have undertaken has not revealed any obvious causes of your symptoms, I highly recommend that you get in touch with us so that we can help you uncover the reasons you are not feeling well. Please see pages 197-198 to learn more.

Can *H pylori* Return?

Unfortunately, it is perfectly feasible that you could have the infection more than once. I know this first hand because I successfully eradicated the infection once, only to find that I picked it up again two years later. Because *H pylori* can be passed from person-to-person and also acquired from contaminated food and water, you can catch it at any time. Contrary to popular belief our bodies do not tend to develop immunity against *H pylori*.

It is very important to ensure that your spouse/partner and children are tested for *H pylori* if you have been diagnosed. If a family member is carrying the infection – whether they have symptoms or not – you may find that it gets back into your body and you're back to square one.

When I felt the symptoms of *H pylori* return, I immediately recommended that my girlfriend should also be tested. Lo and behold, her test came back showing she was *H pylori* positive. Interestingly, she had experienced two occasions of severe stomach pain in the previous twelve months but because the symptoms were sporadic, I didn't associate them with *H pylori*. We both ran stomach cleanses and since that time she has not experienced any digestive symptoms whatsoever and we both feel great.

How Can You Stop H Pylori Coming Back?

Here are the essential steps for maximizing your chances of staying *H pylori*-free:

1. Make sure that all family members are clear. Use the testing available from your doctor. Alternatively, take advantage of our testing services.

2. Ideally, if other family members are infected run the stomach cleanse or medical treatment protocols for each person at the same time.

3. Practice impeccable hygiene – wash dishes and utensils thoroughly and disinfect surfaces.

4. Do not allow pets to lick your face or hands. If they do, wash thoroughly.

5. Eat clean, organically grown food and wash it thoroughly.

6. Follow the *H Pylori Diet* as a preventative measure. If you remain gluten-free and minimize sugar, cow's milk and soy, your immune system will gradually get stronger and you will be far less likely to acquire chronic infections.

7. Stay well hydrated so that your stomach mucosa remains healthy.

8. Reduce your stress levels. Stress lowers immune function.

9. Sleep from 10.30pm-6.30am where possible to allow physical repair, healing and immune function to be optimised.

10. Get plenty of sunlight and exercise because vitamin D is very important for maintaining a healthy immune system and healing the gut.

What If Symptoms Do Not Go Away?

There are several reasons why symptoms may not go away when you run triple therapy or stomach cleanse programmes. These are:

1. *H pylori* bacteria were not completely eradicated.

2. *H pylori* was eradicated successfully but your stomach and intestines have been damaged and need time to heal, just like a cut, burn or wound on your skin needs time to heal. Symptoms can remain during this healing process.

3. You have a yeast/fungal overgrowth that needs to be addressed.

4. You have another digestive infection. This is very common. In fact, when I analysed my lab stats for 2009, I found that 52% of people with *H pylori* also had a parasite, fungal overgrowth or other bacterial problem.

5. Foods that you are still eating are causing you problems. Unfortunately we all have individual reactions against foods. Some people can react against seemingly innocuous foods such as bananas and broccoli. Food allergy testing may be warranted for some people.

If your symptoms do not improve or have worsened following *The H Pylori Diet*, antibiotics and/or the stomach cleanse, please contact my office. We may need to run a more thorough consultation and some individualised lab testing to establish why you're not making the progress we would expect. Don't worry – there is always an answer as to why symptoms are not clearing. Often it's as simple as finding out which foods you are reacting to or the additional digestive infections you have.

Other Digestive Infections

I can't emphasise strongly enough the benefits of running comprehensive stool testing if you have digestive symptoms. As I've gone to great lengths to explain, the majority of 'mysterious' irritable bowel-type symptoms people suffer from are simply the result of something being in the gut that shouldn't be there.

As well as *H pylori*, my colleagues and I see a plethora of different invaders, ranging from bacteria to microscopic parasites and even worms. These parasites and bacterial overgrowths are extremely common but unfortunately, they are hugely underestimated by the medical system. Cast your mind back to the story of Barry Marshall and Robin Warren, who were awarded the Nobel Prize for proving that *H pylori* infection causes ulcers. It took those brilliant guys twenty years to shift the belief of the medical community.

Right now, we face a similar situation with a whole host of other digestive infections. There is no doubt whatsoever that parasites and bacterial overgrowth cause digestive symptoms in millions of people. It's just as easy to pick up these 'bugs' as it is to acquire *H pylori*. I am fortunate enough to see hundreds of lab test results each year and I absolutely guarantee you that *H pylori* is the tip of the iceberg. We have an epidemic of chronic digestive infections that are being completely misdiagnosed as irritable bowel syndrome and people are not receiving the simple testing and treatments they need.

Unless a patient is suffering with extreme digestive pains, vomiting and diarrhoea, it is assumed that parasites can't be present. But time and time again I'm able to help people overcome their symptoms by helping them identify which digestive invaders they have and teaching them how to deal with them. Remember the three sample lab reports from my clients on pages 53-55. They are perfect examples of how hidden chronic digestive infections can lurk and cause a multitude of problems. Ten of the most common digestive 'bugs' I see in my clients' test results are:

✓ *Giardia lamblia*

✓ *Blastocystis hominis* (I had this one)

✓ *Cryptosporidium parvum*

✓ *Dientamoeba fragilis*

✓ *Endolimax nana*

✓ *Trichiura trichuris* (whipworm)

✓ *Ascaris lumbricoides* (roundworm)

✓ *Necator americanus* (hookworm)

✓ *Strongyloides* (threadworm)

✓ *Clostridium difficile*

In addition to these parasitic infections, *Candida albicans* and other yeast and fungal infections are very common and I have also seen cases of opportunistic bacteria such as *Klebsiella, Salmonella, Yersinia, Pseudomonas* and *Vibrio* species. I recommend that you read my book, *What Your Doctor Didn't Tell You About Parasites*. It is currently available in e-book form for you to download. The material teaches you:

✓ Detailed descriptions of the most common human digestive parasites.

✓ Diagrams of the most common parasites.

✓ The vast array of symptoms parasites can create.

✓ How they cause these symptoms.

✓ Why doctors don't acknowledge the problems they cause.

✓ How to identify whether you have them.

✓ How to clear them from your body.

✓ More sample lab reports and case histories, like the ones in this book.

Details on how to order this book as well as how to access our comprehensive lab testing services can be found on pages 197-198 and 202.

How Long Will It Take Before You Feel Well Again?

As much as I would love to be able to look into a crystal ball and provide an answer to this question, it is simply impossible to do so. As you have seen, many factors influence healing time. Some of you may realistically feel better within days of removing gluten from your diet. Some of you might not feel any improvement from this, but you may feel better very quickly when you begin taking the stomach cleanse supplements or triple therapy. Unfortunately some of you may not feel better even if you eradicate *H pylori* because of either having a lot of collateral damage from a long term infection, or the presence of some of the other 'bugs' as previously outlined.

If you have other infections, you may actually feel worse or develop new symptoms when you clear your *H pylori*. In these situations, it is absolutely essential for you to seek professional guidance. The other digestive invaders we see are all capable of causing a huge array of digestive symptoms.

Even where other organisms are not present, it is still possible for healing time to be a little slow, particularly if your stomach and intestinal lining has been damaged by *H pylori* and the likes of gluten. Imagine for a moment having a piece of glass stuck in your finger. If you remove the glass, it doesn't mean that the damage is automatically repaired! The same is true with *H pylori*. Although gut tissue tends to heal quite quickly, the collateral damage resulting from having the infection won't necessarily go away immediately.

It is also important to remember that despite removing some of the key foods that are generically not good for humans, you may still have an individual reaction to seemingly innocuous foods. I've seen amazing turnarounds in clients' health when foods such as innocent as nuts, bananas, eggs and broccoli have been eliminated. We are able to run food allergy and sensitivity testing as part of our service.

How Long Should You Follow The Eating Plan?

It is my recommendation that you adopt the eating strategies in this book for 60-90 days. This allows time for the damaged gut lining to begin healing from the effects of the gluten and other irritating foods.

- If your symptoms improve from removing these foods, my advice is simple: minimise them for the rest of your life. Strict avoidance may not be necessary and if you enjoy eating those foods, a little of them now and again is not likely to hurt you. Nevertheless, use your discretion.

- If removing the foods does not improve your symptoms, I still recommend avoiding them for the initial 60-90 day period, or until you have completed the stomach cleanse because your body may need time to adjust and heal. If your symptoms are still present after 90 days, I implore you to consider running more comprehensive testing to determine why you're not feeling better.

• Once you are symptom-free and assuming the programme works well for you, you may like to reintroduce the problem-foods (namely gluten, milk, soy and sugar) one at a time. By doing this you should be able to gauge whether or not they trigger any symptoms. This may also help you find a tolerance level to those foods. For example, you may find that you can tolerate one slice of toast, but not two.

• Your long term strategy should be to listen to your body's signals. If you eat something and it makes you feel unwell, avoid it. This goes for all foods and beverages.

Closing Comments

H pylori is a major contributor to poor digestive health and because the digestive system is one of the key systems in the body, disruption to its function can prove very detrimental to overall health. You have seen how *H pylori* may cause or contribute to:

• Heartburn
• Acid reflux
• Stomach pain
• Bloating
• Nausea
• Vomiting
• Diarrhoea
• Constipation
• Ulcers
• Stomach cancer
• Skin diseases

- Mood problems
- Fatigue
- Autoimmune conditions such as type I diabetes
- Insulin resistance
- Blood lipid & cholesterol imbalances
- Metabolic Syndrome
- Heart disease
- Strokes

It is therefore essential to take the following steps if you are faced with any of the health challenges listed above:

✓ Make sure you get access to the right testing.

✓ If your doctor won't test you, take matters into your own hands.

✓ If you are infected with *H pylori*, understand that the treatments do not always work, but that there are highly effective alternatives.

✓ Also understand that diet changes can provide significant relief to your symptoms.

✓ Go out of your way to take a retest following treatment but make sure you wait four weeks after completing treatment and do not use the blood test to re-test for *H pylori* as it is completely useless for this purpose.

✓ If family members or those closest to you are experiencing symptoms, get them tested.

Finally, if your symptoms do not resolve and you do not know where to turn, contact my office. We can help you discover why you are not making progress and identify roadblocks such as parasites and food allergies as well as providing detailed health coaching and consultancy.

It is my belief that I should not have needed to write this book. But we have a huge problem in healthcare. Pharmaceutical companies make money by selling drugs. But 'drug-deficiencies' are not the problem. You do not develop symptoms from a lack of drugs and there is always a cause.

I've not only taught you about *H pylori* but also many other possible causes of your symptoms. You now know more about *H pylori*, food sensitivities and the many other digestive infections than 99% of the doctors in the Western world so please share this information with as many people as you can.

It is my hope that this information has been of great help to you. I also dearly hope that you can go away and apply the principles I have taught so that your symptoms are resolved quickly. You are now on a journey and I truly hope it takes you to your perfect destination, whatever that might be for you.

Wishing you all the very best,

Dave Hompes

Dave Hompes.

Comprehensive Digestive Testing In Your Home

The GI Effects Comprehensive Stool Test by Metametrix

If you are:

✓ Unsure of what is causing your symptoms.

✓ Experiencing difficulty in getting your doctor to authorise testing.

✓ Not resolving your symptoms despite diet changes and treatment.

✓ Looking to re-test to check that *H pylori* has gone...

...it is possible for you to run testing in the comfort of your own home. Stool testing kits can be mailed to your home where you complete the sample and simply mail it back to the lab for analysis.

The benefits of comprehensive stool testing are:

✓ Identify the cause of your digestive symptoms.

✓ Discover why you are feeling tired.

✓ Find out why you have skin problems.

✓ Receive information that allows you to remove the guesswork follow a laser-focused recovery protocol.

✓ Shortcut the waiting process that is often involved with medical testing.

✓ Speed up healing time.

✓ Save money on medical treatments and supplements that don't work.

✓ Expert interpretation and explanation of your results.

The testing can identify more than 80 different digestive markers and uses a cutting edge DNA PCR amplification technique to identify micro-organisms, which is up to five thousand times more sensitive in finding certain parasites than standard stool microscopy tests:

✓ 23 different digestive parasites (including *Giardia, Cryptosporidium, Blastocystis,* amoebae, worms such as hookworm, pinworm and whipworm, threadworm.

✓ Countless opportunistic bacteria, including *Salmonella, Vibrio, Staphylococcus aureas, Yersinia, Klebsiella, Aeromonas.*

✓ Pathogenic bacteria including *H pylori, C. difficile, E. coli,* and *Campylobacter.*

✓ Yeast & fungal overgrowth

✓ Sensitivity of bacterial and fungal overgrowth to pharmaceutical and botanical agents.

✓ Your balance of 'good' or 'friendly' bacteria.

✓ Gluten sensitivity

✓ 'Collateral damage' such as inflammation, protective chemicals called short chain fatty acid levels.

✓ Presence of blood and mucus in stools.

✓ Digestive enzyme levels.

✓ Digestion and absorption of proteins, fats and vegetable fibres.

✓ Professional laboratory interpretation, programme design, consultancy and ongoing support.

For more information, including sample reports, a free hour-long teleseminar recording, patient and interpretive guides and more, please visit: **www.H-Pylori-Symptoms.com/h-pylori-testing**

Alternatively call our offices on **0800 310 2121** (UK); or **+44 7856 269 750** (International)

Claim Your 50% Discount & Free Lessons

The Health Freedom Secrets Online Programme

The *H Pylori Diet* programme is an advanced tool for helping you achieve your health-related goals. But just like any book it has its limitations. We heard from a lot of people that they were a little overwhelmed by the information and struggled to adjust their routines to include all the recommendations.

So I created a solution to this problem: it's called *Health Freedom Secrets*!

The *Health Freedom Secrets* programme is the most comprehensive - but also the most convenient and easy to follow - health programme I know of.

This ten-week life changing programme allows me to coach you through the process of implementing all the tips and strategies included in this book step-by-step, at a fraction of the cost of working with my consultants individually. Let me take you by the hand and ensure that you maximise the benefits of this information.

Week by week, *Health Freedom Secrets* takes you through ten specifically designed lessons that teach you everything you could ever need to know about diet and nutrition. In fact, I've had qualified nutritionists tell me that this programme taught them more practical diet and nutrition nuggets than their entire three year nutrition degree!

Each week you are sent an email with access to a new lesson that contains a presentation, audio recording, Action Guide and Resource Guide. The goal is for you to implement the information on a week-by-week basis so that that it is easy to follow and does not create more stress for you.

There's an introductory lesson, followed by presentations, action and resource guides covering:

✓ Lesson One – The true importance of water and hydration and why many symptoms diseases are just your body's many cries for water.

✓ Lesson Two – Macronutrients (fats, proteins & carbohydrates): the real building blocks of health and why consideration of these is far more important than vitamins and minerals.

✓ Lesson Three – Breakfast: how to perfect the toughest meal of the day!

✓ Lesson Four – Lunches: how to get a great lunch despite a healthy lifestyle!

✓ Lesson Five – Dinner, Snacks and the critical need for good blood sugar control!

✓ Lesson Six – Gluten and grains: the true story of how these dietary mainstays can destroy your health and how to make sure that doesn't happen to you!

✓ Lesson Seven – Milk: the deadly poison: how you are tricked into believing that you need to consume cow's milk to be healthy and what you can do instead!

✓ Lesson Eight – The critical difference between raw food and cooked food and how to optimise the raw food in your diet.

✓ Lesson Nine – How alcohol, sugar and artificial sweeteners affect your health and how you can use replacements to minimise your exposure.

✓ Lesson Ten – How to make sure you digest and absorb the food you eat.

There are also four bonus lessons on specific and important topics that help to 'supercharge' the programme:

✓ Bonus One – The truth about food allergies and how you can run food allergy testing at home that costs absolutely nothing!

✓ Bonus Two – How to truly individualise your diet using the concept of Metabolic Typing.

✓ Bonus Three – Is "Organic" food a rip-off? How to source the very finest fresh food that boosts your body and protects your environment!

✓ Bonus Four – How to read food labels so that you are not deceived by clever marketing thereby enabling you to make informed decisions about what you put in your mouth.

You can download all the lessons, add them to an MP3 player or to a CD so that you can consume the information when and where it suits you.

To make it even easier for you to follow the programme, *Health Freedom Secrets* also comes with a complete Shopping Tips, Menu and Recipe Guide, especially written by qualified chef and health coach, Karen Maidment. In fact, you get a free copy of the *H Pylori Digest-Ease Recipe & Cookbook* as part of the programme. This guide is packed full of gluten, soy and milk-free recipes and meal ideas to make sure that you have an almost endless supply of tasty but utterly healthy meals.

For more detailed information simply visit **www.HealthFreedomSecrets.com/special.**

Your discount coupon is **FMS030275**

Simply enter this discount code where prompted to receive your 50% discount!

What Your Doctor Didn't Tell You About Parasites

E-Book – available as an instant download

In order to overcome your symptoms, you simply must know what's causing them in the first place. Unfortunately 95% of doctors won't even think about testing you for hidden digestive infections such as parasites. Other digestive infections can cause or contribute to exactly the same symptoms as *Helicobacter pylori*. The infections can be classified into three main categories: parasites, bacteria and yeast/fungi.

What Your Doctor Didn't Tell You About Parasites is en e-book that you can download instantly onto your computer to learn about the common digestive parasites that cause a multitude of day-to-day symptoms both inside and outside the digestive system. The TOP TEN digestive 'bugs' are discussed, along with relevant pharmaceutical and botanical/herbal programmes that can be used to remove them.

It also contains an educational section on other common bacteria that are known to cause chronic symptoms and that we see regularily in client lab reports. These bacteria include *Salmonella, Vibrio, E.coli, C.difficile* and *Staphylococcus aureus* (strains of which are known as MRSA).

This e-book is a *must read f*or anyone who is struggling to overcome *H pylori* or who wants to overcome mysterious symptoms such as IBS, fatigue, sleep, skin and mood problems.

To order your copy now visit
www.H-Pylori-Symptoms.com/parasite-book

Every effort has been made to ensure that the information within this book is accurate and up to date. However I acknowledge that research into the area of *H pylori* and, indeed in the wider area of general digestive health is continuously expanding our knowledge. As such, this book is likely to be updated on an annual basis.

To see a full bibliography and reference list I invite you to visit the web page below:

www.H-Pylori-Symptoms.com/h-pylori-studies

Here you will find a multitude of books and studies to support the information presented in this book. Should your physician question the materials within *The H Pylori Diet* I recommend that you direct him to this reference list.

If you are interested in learning more about *H pylori* on a technical level, or require further evidence to present to your doctor I highly recommend that you visit **www.Helicobacter.org**. This is the website of the European Helicobacter Study Group and it is the richest source of information on *H pylori* anywhere.

References

Welcome to the reference list and bibliography in support of the material presented in this book. This is not an exhaustive list of H pylori references and resources. For additional research findings I highly recommend that you visit **www.Helicobacter.org**, home of the European Helicobacter study group and medical journal.

H Pylori, Other Helicobacters & Infection In Humans

Guerreiro et al. Detection of *Helicobacter pylori* DNA in the Oral Cavity of a Portuguese Population. *Helicobacter* 2003 (A06.26); 8: 339-493.

Timmins, W. Resolving Chronic Stress Related Disorders. *Biohealth Diagnostics DVD Set*, 2006 (Dr. Timmins discusses isolating *H pylori* in semen samples).

Salmanian et al. Amplification of babA and Urease genes of *Helicobacter pylori* from Oral, Gastric and Vaginal Yeasts. *Helicobacter* 2006 (A04.08); 11: 321-415.

Labropoulou et al. *Helicobacter pylori* Identified Immunohistochemically in Resected Gallbladder Mucosa and in the remains of Cholesterol Gallstones a Case Report. *Helicobacter* 2003 (A13.06); 8: 339-493.

Helmy et al. Identification of *Helicobacter* sp. in Bile and Laparoscopicly Resected Gallbladder Tissue from Egyptians with Chronic Calcular Cholecystitis. *Helicobacter* 2007 (P037); 12: 379-476.

Bielawski et al. Detection of *Helicobacter* Species in Liver Tissue of Polish Patients with Chronic Liver Disease by PCR-DGGE and Sequence Analysis. *Helicobacter* 2005 (A15.06); 10: 458-556.

Sturegard et al. Detection of *Helicobacter* Species in Colon Biopsies. *Helicobacter.* 2003 (A14.09); 8: 339-493.

Labropoulou et al. Do hyperplastic polyps of the colorectum represent an extragastric reservoir for Helicobacter pylori infection? *Helicobacter* 2004 (A08.08); 9: 487-604.

Labropoulou et al. *Helicobacter pylori* in Tonsil Tissue of Greeks. *Helicobacter* 2003 (A06.18); 8: 339-493.

Labropoulou et al. *Helicobacter pylori* colonisation in palatine salivary glands. *Helicobacter* 2004 (A04.022); 9: 487-604.

www.infek.lu.se/bakt/english/helicobacter

Distribution & Transmission of *H Pylori*

Fleming, SL. PhD, 2007. *Helicobacter pylori*. Chelsea House Publications.

Graham, K. S. M.D & Graham, D.Y. M.D, 2002. *Contemporary Diagnosis and Management of H. pylori-Associated Gastrointestinal Disease*. Handbooks in Healthcare Co.

Kivi *et al*. Concordance of *Helicobacter pylori* Strains Within Families. *Helicobacter* 2003 (A06.04); 8: 339-493

Wai-Keung Leung, Joseph J. Y. Sung, Thomas K. W. Ling, Kris L. K. Siu and Augustine F. B. Cheng. Use of Chopsticks for Eating and *Helicobacter pylori* Infection. *JDig Dis Sci*. 1999 44 (6): 1173-1176

Kafritsa *et al*. H. pylori in children's dental plaque: Correlation with the *H pylori* Infection status of their parents. *Helicobacter* 2002; 7: A32.

Weyermann *et al*. The Mother as Intrafamilial Source of *Helicobacter pylori* Infection: A Prospective Birth Cohort. *Helicobacter* 2005 (A04.06); 10: 458-556.

Cunha *et al*, 2002. Prevalence and risk factors associated to *Helicobacter pylori* infection among natives from Western Amazon rainforest, Brazil. *Helicobacter*. 2002; 7: A6.18.

Azevedo *et al*, 2005. Factors Affecting the Adhesion of Water-Stressed *Helicobacter pylori* to plumbing Materials. *Helicobacter* 2005 (A04.13); 10: 458-556.

Garcia-Amado *et al*. Isolation of *Helicobacter* spp. from Seawater, Plankton and Oysters from Areas of the Caribbean Sea Subject to Faecal Contamination. *Helicobacter* 2005 (A15.15); 10: 458-556.

Puiqueres *et al*. Rapid detection of *Helicobacter pylori* in vegetables irrigated with contaminated water. *Helicobacter* 2004 (A04.18); 9: 487-604.

www.naturalchoices.co.uk/Salmonella-levels-over-5x-higher?id_mot=7

Liebowitz M. Via Personal Communication with Dr. Dan Kalish regarding eggs as a possible transmission route for *H pylori*.

Hunt, R.H., & Tytgat, G.N.J., 1998 *Helicobacter pylori: Basic Mechanisms to Clinical Cure*.

Imamura et al, 2003. Cockroaches can be possible carriers of *Helicobacter pylori*. *Helicobacter* 2003 (A06.19); 8: 339-493.

Tytgat GNJ. Endoscopic transmission of *Helicobacter pylori*. Aliment Pharmacol Ther. 1995; (9) Supp 2: 105-110.

Gueneau et al. Detection of *Helicobacter* sp. in sharks, bivalve molluscs, corals and water filtrates from the Caribbean Sea suggests that infection is common and transmission occurs through water. *Helicobacter* 2003 (A06.10); 8: 339-493.

Citelly et al, 2002. *Helicobacter pylori* in animals is of human origin: studies in monkeys sheep and cats. *Helicobacter* 2002; 7: A31.

Gosciniak et al. Prevalence of Anti-*Helicobacter* spp. Antibodies in Dogs. *Helicobacter* 2007 (P038); 12: 379-476.

Van den Bulck *et al*. Prevalence of *Helicobacter felis*, H *bizzozeronii* and H *salomonis* in Dogs and Cats. *Helicobacter* 2003 (A09.04); 8: 339-493.

Siavoshi et al, 2007. Animals Harbouring Yeast Might Play a Role in Transmission of *Helicobacter pylori*. *Helicobacter* 2007 (P137); 12: 379-476.

Cartagenes VD *et al*. *Helicobacter pylori* in children and association with Cag-A strains in mother-child transmission in the Brazilian Amazon region. *Rev Soc Bras Med Trop*. 2009; 42:298-302.

Yucel O *et al*. The factors associated with asymptomatic carriage of *Helicobacter pylori* in children and their mothers living in three socio-economic settings. *Jpn J Infect Dis*. 2009; 62:120-4.

Roma E *et al*. Intrafamilial spread of *Helicobacter pylori* infection in Greece. *J Clin Gastroenterol*. 2009; 43:711-15.

Alexander. C. Ford & Anthony T.R. Axon. Epidemiology of *Helicobacter pylori* Infection and Public Health Implications. *Helicobacter* 2010; 15 (Suppl.1) 1-6.

Adams BL *et al*. Survival of *Helicobacter pylori* in a natural freshwater environment. *Appl Env Mic*. 2003; 69(12): 7462-66.

Megraud F & Broutet N. Epidemioloigy, acquisition and transmission of *Helicobacter pylori*. *Rev Prat* 2000; Sep 1; 50(13):1417-7.

Van Duynhoven YT & de Jonge R. Transmission of *Helicobacter pylori*: a role for food? *Bull World Health Org*. 2001; 79(5): 455-60.

Gyorgy Miklos Buzas. Gastric tubes as vectors of *Helicobacter pylori* transmission. *Medical Hypotheses*. 2010; 75(1), 47-49.

Symptoms & Conditions Associated With *H Pylori* Infection

Various

It is well established that *H pylori* causes gastritis, duodenitis and peptic ulcers. Because information on this specific topic is widespread, I have not included many references. The single reference below is the latest review article written on how *H pylori* infection leads to these conditions.

De Vries AC & Kuipers, EJ. *Helicobacter pylori* infection and non-malignant diseases. *Helicobacter* 2010; 15 (Suppl.1) 29-33.

Anaemia

Sarker *et al*. Anti-*Helicobacter pylori* Therapy Improves Iron Status and Gastric Acid Output in Young Bangladeshi Women with H. pylori-Associated Hypochloridia and Iron Deficiency Anaemia. *Helicobacter* 2006 (A06.01); 11: 321-415.

Sarker et al. Serum Ferritin, Haemoglobin, Soluble Transferrin Receptor and *Helicobacter pylori* Infection in Peri-Urban Community Children in Bangladesh. *Helicobacter* 2005 (A09.06); 10: 458-556.

Munoz-Codoceo. Iron deficiency anaemia in paediatric patients with *Helicobacter pylori* infection. *Helicobacter* 2004 (A09.21); 9: 487-604.

Russo-Mancuso *et al*. Iron Deficiency Anaemia as the only sign of Infection with *Helicobacter pylori*: A Report of 9 Paediatric cases. *Int J. Haemat.* 78: 429-431.

Bronchitis

Roussos *et al*. *Helicobacter pylori* Seroprevalence in patients with Chronic Bronchitis. *Journal of Gastroenterology*. 2002; 37:332-335.

Colitis

Pena *et al*. *Helicobacter hepaticus*-induced Colitis is diminished by coinfection with *Lactobacillus*. *Helicobacter* 2003 (A08.03); 8: 339-493.

Cancer (Extragastric – i.e. Outside Stomach))

Rokkas *et al*, 2006. Meta-analyses on the Relationship between *Helicobacter pylori* infection and Extra-gastric GI cancers. *Helicobacter* 2006 (A07.13); 11: 321-415.

Shmuely *et al*. *Helicobacter pylori* CagA Status and Colorectal Cancer. *Helicobacter* 2003 (A10.09); 8: 339-493.

Wohrer S et al. *Helicobacter pylori* and pancreatic cancer. A working hypothesis from epidemiological studies. *J. Pancreas* (Online) 2003; 4(4): 163-164.

Nilsson *et al*. *Helicobacter* Species in the Pancreas, Stomach and Duodenum of Patients with Pancreas Cancer. *Helicobacter* 2003 (A13.04); 8: 339-493

Crohn's Disease

Zerbib *et al*. Prevalence of Entero-Hepatic *Helicobacters* in Crohn's Disease: Preliminary study. *Helicobacter* 2003 (A09.12); 8: 339-493.

Oliveira *et al*. Crohn's Disease and *Helicobacter* Species in the Intestinal Mucosa. *Helicobacter* 2003 (A14.04); 8: 339-493.

Halitosis / Bad Breath

Lerardi *et al*. Halitosis and *Helicobacter Pylori*. A Possible Relationship. *Dig Dis Sci*. 1998 (43); 12: 2733-2737.

Skin Disease (Rosacea, Urticaria, ITP, Prurigo, Pruritis, etc)

Hernando-Harder, AC. *et al*. *H pylori* and Dermatologic Disease. *Eur Journal Dermatol* 2009; 19(5): 431-44.

The above paper is an excellent review article that summarises the findings of many studies conducted on the relationship between *H pylori* and skin diseases.

Novak *et al*. Elevated levels of anti-Helicobacter pylori antibodies in Henoch-Schonlein purpura. *Autoimmunity*. 2003 Aug; 36(5): 307-11.

Gasbarrini *et al,* 1998. Helicobacter pylori Eradication Ameliorates Primary Raynaud's Phenomenon.

Figura *et al*. Helicobacter pylori infection and rosacea: an immunoproteomic study of a case. *Helicobacter* 2004 (A08.14); 9: 487-604.

Di Campli *et al*. Beneficial Effects of *Helicobacter pylori* Eradication on Chronic Idiopathic Urticaria. *Dig Dis Sci*. 1998; 43(6):1226-1229.

H Pylori & Heart Disease

Huang B, *et al*. Cag-A positive *Helicobacter pylori* strains enhanced coronary atherosclerosis by increasing serum OcLDL and HsCRP in patients with coronary heart disease. *Dig Dis Sci*. 2010 May 26 [Epub ahead of print].

Niccoli G *et al*. Coronary atherosclerotic burden in patients with infection by Cag-A-positive strains of *Helicobacter pylori*. *Coron Artery Dis*. 2010 Jun; 21 (4): 217-21.

Shmuely H, *et al*. Association of Cag-A+ *Helicobacter pylori* infection with aortic atheroma. *Atherosclerosis*. 2005 Mar; 179(1):127-32.

Zhang S *et al*. Cytotoxin-associated gene-A-seropositive virulent strains of *Helicobacter pylori* and atherosclerotic diseases: a systematic review. *Chin Med J*. 2008 May 20; 121(10):946-51.

Pasceri V, *et* al. Virulent strains of *Helicobacter pylori* and vascular diseases: a meta-analysis. *Am Heart J.* 2006 Jun; 151(6):1215-22.

Gunn M, *et al.* Significant association of Cag-A+ *Helicobacter pylori* strains with risk of premature myocardial infarction. *Heart.* 2000 Sep; 84(3): 267-71.

Kowalski M. *Helicobacter pylori* infection in coronary artery disease: influence of *H Pylori* eradication on coronary artery lumen after percutaneous transluminal coronary angioplasty. The detection of *H pylori* specific DNA in human coronary atherosclerotic plaque. *J Physiol Pharmacol.* 2001 Aug; 52(1Suppl 1):3-31.

Association of Helicobacter pylori infection with systemic inflammation and endothelial dysfunction in healthy male subjects. *J Am Coll Cardiol.* 2005; 45:1219-1222.

Bajenov *et al.* *Helicobacter pylori* Infection of the Patients with Ischemic Heart Disease. *Helicobacter* 2005 (A05.27); 10: 458-556.

Franceschi *et al.* Atherosclerotic Burden in Patients with Infection Sustained by CagA-Positive Strains of *Helicobacter pylori.* *Helicobacter* 2007 (AW1.07); 12: 379-476.

Choi *et al.* Association of *Helicobacter pylori* Infection with Cardiovascular Risk Factors in Korean Adults who were Diagnosed with Coronary Heart Disease. *Helicobacter* 2006 (A05.15); 11: 321-415.

Sperduti *et al,* 2006. Evaluation of Sub clinical Vascular Alterations in *Helicobacter pylori Positive* Patients. *Helicobacter* 2006 (A06.10); 11: 321-415.

Franceschi *et al.* Virulent Strains of *Helicobacter pylori* in Patients with Stable and Unstable Angina Pectoris. *Helicobacter* 2005 (A08.09); 10: 458-556.

Gabrielli *et al.* Cag-A Positive Cytotoxic *H pylori* Strains: a Link between Plaque Instability and Atherosclerotic Stroke? *Helicobacter* 2003 (A14.05); 8: 339-493.

Oral Health & Heart Disease

Cesar de Oliveira. Toothbrushing, inflammation and the risk of cardiovascular disease: results from Scottish Health Survey. *BMJ.* 2010; 340:c2451.

H *Pylori* & C-Reactive Protein (CRP)

CRP is what is known as an acute phase protein and is produced by the body in response to inflammation, including the inflammation caused by *H* pylori, other digestive infections and the ingestion of foods such as gluten. CRP a biomarker for increased heart-disease risk.

Ishida Y *et al.* Significant association between *Helicobacter pylori* infection and serum C-reactive protein. *Int J Med Sci.* 2008; 5:224-229.

Bunch TJ *et al*. Frequency of *Helicobacter pylori* seropositivity and C-reactive protein increase in atrial fibrillation in patients undergoing coronary angiography. *Am J Cardiol*. 2008 Mar 15; 101(6):848-51.

Kanbay M, *et al*. Does eradication of *Helicobacter pylori* infection help normalise serum lipid and CRP levels? *Dig Dis Sci*. 2005 Jul;50(7): 1228-31.

H Pylori & Blood Pressure, Insulin Resistance & Type II Diabetes

Migneco A *et al*. Eradication of *Helicobacter pylori* infection improves blood pressure values in patients affected by hypertension. *Helicobacter*. 2003 Dec; 8(6): 585-9.

Manolakis AC *et al*. Increased fetuin A levels in *Helicobacter pylori* infection: a missing link between *H pylori* and insulin resistance? *Diabetologia*. 2010. Published online at Springerlink.com.

Gen R, *et al*. Effect of *Helicobacter pylori* eradication on insulin resistance, serum lipids and low-grade inflammation. *South Med J*. 2010 Mar;103(3): 190-6.

Longo-Mbenza B *et al*. Prevention of the metabolic syndrome, insulin resistance and the atherosclerotic diseases in Africans infected by *Helicobacter pylori* infection and treated by antibiotics. *Int J Cardiol*. 2007 Oct 18:121(3):229-38.

Eshraghian, A *et al*. *Helicobacter pylori* infection as a risk factor for insulin resistance. *Dig Dis Sci*. 2009; 54(9):1966-70.

Wang SZ, Shi YN, Zhao J, Wang ZD Effects of *Helicobacter pylori* on blood glucose fluctuations in type 2 diabetic patients. Zhonghua Yi Xue Za Zhi. 2009 Apr 14; 89(14):958-61.

Gunji T *et al*. *Helicobacter pylori* infection significantly increases insulin resistance in the asymptomatic Japanese population. *Helicobacter.* 2009 Oct; 14(5):144-50.

Aydemir S. *et al*. The Effect of *Helicobacter pylori* on insulin resistance. *Dig Dis Sci.*2005 Nov;50(11):2090-3.

Gunji, T *et al*. *Helicobacter pylori* infection is significantly associated with metabolic syndrome in the Japanese population. *Am J Gastroenterol*. 2008 Dec; 103(12):3005-10.

Aslan M, *et al*. Insulin resistance in *H pylori* infection and its association with oxidative stress. *World J Gastroenterol*. 2006 Nov 14; 12(42):6865-8.

Satoh H, *et al*. *Helicobacter pylori* infection is a significant risk for modified lipid profile in Japanese male subjects. *J Atherscler Thromb*. 2010 Oct 27; 17(10): 1041-8.

Aydemir *et al*. The Effect of *Helicobacter pylori* on Insulin Resistance. *Dig Dis Sci.* 2005; (11): 2090-2093.

Vitamin B12 & Folic Acid Deficiency

Ciok *et al*. *Helicobacter pylori* Eradication and Serum Level of Homocysteine and Folic Acid – 1 Year Intervention Study. *Helicobacter* 2006 (A08.01); 11: 321-415.

Queiroz *et al*. The effect of *Helicobacter pylori* eradication on plasma vitamin B12 and homocysteine levels in elderly patients. *Helicobacter* 2004 (A08.04); 9: 487-604.

Sipponen *et al*. *H pylori* Related Atrophic Gastritis is a Common Cause of low Vitamin B12 and High Homocysteine in Serum in an Elderly Male Population. *Helicobacter* 2003 (A07.01); 8: 339-493.

Kaptan *et al*. *Helicobacter pylori* – is it a novel causative agent in vitamin B12 deficiency? *Arch Intern Med.* 2000; (160): 1349-1353.

Carmel *et al*. *Helicobacter pylori* Infection and Food-Cobalamin Malabsorption. *Dig Dis Sci.* 1994; (39) 2: 309-314.

Lewerin *et al*. Serum biomarkers for atrophic gastritis and antibodies against *Helicobacter pylori* in the elderly: Implications for vitamin B12, folic acid and iron status and response to oral vitamin therapy. *Scandinavian Journal of Gastroenterology*. 2008; (9):1050-56.

H Pylori & Low Stomach Acid

Hayakawa *et al*. Role of *Helicobacter pylori* infection on delayed gastric liquid emptying in gastric ulcers. *Helicobacter* 2004 (A06.03); 9: 487-604.

Hoffman *et al*. Rabbit and Ferret Parietal Cell Inhibition by *Helicobacter* Species. *Dig Dis Sci.* 1995; (40)1: 147-152.

Helicobacter and Gallstones

Belzer *et al*. Urease-induced Calcium Precipitation by Bile-Resistant *Helicobacter* Species ay Initiate Gallstone Formation. *Helicobacter* 2006 (A17.01); 11: 321-415.

Abu Al-Soud *et al*. Prevalence of *Helicobacter* and Other Bacteria in Bile and Gallbladder of Kosovan Patients with Chronic Cholecystitis in Correlation to Age, Gender and Urban-rural Differences. *Helicobacter* 2006 (A17.05); 11: 321-415.

Govorun *et al*. *Helicobacter* Species Found in Gallbladder Stones. *Helicobacter* 2002; 7: A74.

Apostolov *et al*. Link Between *Helicobacter* and Chronic Gallbladder Disease. *Helicobacter* 2003 (A13.07); 8: 339-493

H Pylori & The Liver / Hepatitis C (HCV)

Queiroz *et al.* Detection of *Helicobacter pylori* in the Liver of Patients with Different Aetiologies of Hepatic diseases. *Helicobacter* 2007 (AW2.08); 12: 379-476

Candelli *et al.Helicobacter pylori* Infection in HCV-Related Chronic Liver Disease & Thrombocytopenia. *Helicobacter* 2005 (A11.19); 10: 458-556.

Giannini *et al, Helicobacter pylori* Infection is Associated with Greater Impairment of Cytochrome P-450 Liver Metabolic Activity in Anti-HCV Positive Cirrhotic Patients. *Dig Dis Sci.* 2003; 48(4): 802-808.

Kosunen *et al.* The Effect of Eradication Therapy for *Helicobacter pylori* Infection on the Incidence of Gastric and Other Cancers. *Helicobacter* 2006 (A07.08); 11: 321-415.

Migraine & Headaches

Di Bastiani *et al.* Improvement of Migraine after *H pylori* Eradication. *Helicobacter* 2004 (A08.15); 9: 487-604.

Gabrielli *et al.* Beneficial Effects of *Helicobacter pylori* Eradication on Migraine: a 12-Month follow-up study. *Journal of Headache Pain.* 2001 2):39-43.

Osteoporosis

Figura *et al. H pylori* Infection, risk of osteoporosis and systemic levels of estrogens. *Helicobacter* 2004 (A08.09); 9: 487-604.

Figura *et al.* Possible influence of *H pylori* infection on parameters of bone reabsorption in male patients with osteoporosis. *Helicobacter* 2002; 7: A78.

Fibromyalgia

Akkaya et al. Helicobacter seroposotivity in fibromyalgia syndrome. Clin Rheumatol. 2010 Dec 1 [Epub ahead of print].

Pancreatitis

Rieder *et al.* Is *Helicobacter pylori* Gastritis a Risk Factor for Chronic Pancreatitis in Mongolian Gerbils? *Helicobacter* 2006 (A06.02); 11: 321-415.

Naumovski-Mihalic *et al. Helicobacter pylori* Infection as A Cause of Acute Pancreatitis: Fact or Fiction? *Helicobacter* 2006 (A08.09); 11: 321-415.

Lucca et al, 2004. Alcoholic chronic pancreatitis, duodenal ulcer and *H pylori* infection. *Helicobacter* 2004 (A04.21); 9: 487-604.

Parkinson's Disease

Bjarnason *et al.* Double-blind, placebo-controlled trial of eradication of *Helicobacter pylori* in idiopathic Parkinsonism. *Helicobacter* 2004 (A08.07); 9: 487-604.

Pietroiusti *et al*. Short and Long Term Effects of *Helicobacter pylori* Eradication on Clinical Response to L-dopa in Parkinson's Disease Patients. *Helicobacter* 2004 (A08.10); 9: 487-604.

Sperm

Capitani *et al*, 2007. Sperm Characteristics in Patients with Reproductive Disorders Infected by CagA-Positive and CagA-Negative *Helicobacter pylori* Strains. *Helicobacter* 2007 (P049); 12: 379-476

Autoimmine Thyroiditis (Thyroid Disorders)

Figura *et al*, 2005. *Helicobacter pylori* Infection and Autoimmune Diseases: Prevalence of Infection in Patients with Hashimoto's Thyroiditis and Alignment of Thyroid Hormones with H. pylori Proteins. *Helicobacter* 2005 (A08.08); 10: 458-556.

Sykora *et al*. The Prevalence of *Helicobacter pylori* infection in Juvenile Lymphocytic Thyroiditis in Childhood and Its Role in the Development of Autoimmunity. *Helicobacter* 2007 (P145); 12: 379-476.

Cavallaro et al, 2007. Is *Helicobacter pylori* Infection related to Body Atrophic Gastritis in Patients Affected by Autoimmune Thyroid Disease? *Helicobacter* 2007 (P189); 12: 379-476.

Type I Diabetes (Insulin-Dependent Diabetes Mellitus)

Ojetti et al, 2005. *Helicobacter pylori* Reinfection in Insulin-Dependent Diabetes Mellitus Patients: A 5-Year Follow-Up. *Helicobacter* 2005 (A04.05); 10: 458-556.

Naumovski-Mihalic *et al*. Eradication of *Helicobacter pylori* Infection in Patients with Diabetes Mellitus. *Helicobacter* 2003 (A14.21); 8: 339-493.

Morning Sickness In Pregnant Women

Michopoulos et al. Helicobacter pylori Seropositivity influences the time of starting as well as the frequency of Vomiting in Pregnancy. *Helicobacter* 2003 (A18.01); 8: 339-493

Shirin *et al*. Positive Serology for *Helicobacter pylori* & Vomiting in the pregnancy. *Arch Gynecol Obstet*. 2004: (270): 10-14.

Medical Treatment For *H Pylori*

Gaby, A. R. *Helicobacter pylori* Eradication: are there alternatives to antibiotics? *Altern Med Rev.* 2001 6 (4): 355-366

Graham, K. S. M.D & Graham, D.Y. M.D, 2002. *Contemporary Diagnosis and Management of H. pylori-Associated Gastrointestinal Disease.* Handbooks in Healthcare Co.

Fleming, S.L. Ph.D, 2007. *Helicobacter pylori.* Chelsea House Publications.

Usta *et al.* Comparison of the Short and Long Term *Helicobacter pylori* Treatment Protocols in Children. *Helicobacter.* 2007 (P065); 12: 379-476

Torres *et al.* Simultaneous colonisation with multiple quacispecies and multiple strains of *Helicobacter pylori* in different regions of the human stomach. *Helicobacter* 2002; 7: A11.

Graham, D. and Shiotani, A. 2008. New Concepts of Resistance in the Treatment of *Helicobacter pylori. Nature Clinical Practice Gastro & Hep.*

Egan *et al, Treatment of Helicobacter pylori. Helicobacter.* 2007; Vol 12; Supp 1, Oct: 31-37.

Uygun *et al.* Sequential Treatment of *Helicobacter pylori* in Patients with Non-ulcer Dyspepsia. *Helicobacter.* 2007 (QW8.06); 12: 379-476

Uygun *et al.* The Efficacy of Bismuth Containing Quadruple Therapy as a First-Line Treatment Option for *Helicobacter pylori. Helicobacter.* 2007 (P067); 12: 379-476

Saltik-Temizel *et al.* Second-Line *Helicobacter pylori* Therapy Eradication Failure in Children. *Helicobacter.* 2007 (P075); 12: 379-476.

Wuppenhorst *et al.* Management of *H pylori* Resistance: Lessons from the First Multivariate Data Analysis of the German Sentinel Study ResiNet. *Helicobacter.* 2007 (P056); 12: 379-476.

O'Connor A. *et al.* Treatment of *Helicobacter pylori* infection 2010. *Helicobacter* 2010; 15 (Suppl.1) 46-52.

Garcia, TG *et al.* High prevalence of Clarithromycin resistance and cag-A, vac-A, ice2 and Bab-A genotypes of *Helicobacter pylori* infection. *J Clin Microb.* 2010 Nov; 48(11): 4266-4268.

"Doctor's Knowledge Article"

www.hormoneandlongevitycenter.com/doctorsknowledge

H Pylori and Yeast / Fungal Problems (Candida)

Siavoshi *et al.* Yeasts of the Oral Cavity Are the Reservoirs of Helicobacter pylori. *Helicobacter.* 2003 (A06.10); 8: 339-493.

Salmanian *et al.* Detection of H. pylori-specific gene in the oral yeasts. *Helicobacter* 2004 (A04.27); 9: 487-604.

Salmanian et al, 2007. Does Oral Yeast Serve as the Host for Other Helicobacter Species? *Helicobacter.* 2007 (W2.07); 12: 379-476.

Latifi-Navid *et al.* Detection of Helicobacter pylori and Yeast in Biopsy Cultures. *Helicobacter.* 2007 (P011); 12: 379-476

Lazebnik *et al.* Role of Helicobacter pylori in Protection from Intestinal Candidosis. *Helicobacter.* 2005 (A08.07); 10: 458-556.

The H Pylori Diet – Food Recommendation References

Gluten

O'Bryan, T. Unlocking The Mystery of Wheat and Gluten Sensitivity. 2006: DVD.

O'Bryan, T. Gluten Sensitivity & Celiac Disease. One-day workshop, London - March 2011.

Green P and Jones R. 2006. *Celiac Disease: A Hidden Epidemic*. Collins.

Braly J and Hoggan MA. 2002. *Dangerous Grains*. Avery.

Cow's Milk

Cohen R. Milk: *The Deadly Poison*.

www.RealMilk.com

Getoff, DJ and McAfee, M. The Whole Truth About Milk. 2007 – DVD.

Soy

Kayla Daniel *The Whole Soy Story*. 2007. New Trends Publishing.

Cooking & Food Preparation

Fallon S and Enig M.1999. *Nourishing Traditions*. New Trends Publishing.

Caveglia, R. *Real Food, Real Fast* (appears to be out of print).

Blood Sugar Balance

Schwarzbein D and Deville N. 1999. *The Schwarzbein Principle: The Truth Sbout Losing Weight, Being Healthy, and Feeling Younger*. Health Communications Inc.

Schwarzbein D and Brown M. 2002. *The Schwarzbein Principle II: The Transition*. Health Communications Inc.

Fat and Cholesterol

Enig, M. Know Your Fats. 2000. Bethseda Press.

Smith J. 2009. *$29 Billion Reasons to Lie About Cholesterol: Making Profit By Turning Healthy People into Patients*. Matador.

Water & Hydration

Batmanghelidj F *Your Body's Many Cries for Water*. Falls Church, VA: Global Health Solutions, Inc.

Fox, M. *Healthy Water*. Portsmouth, NH: Healthy Water Research 1990, 1998 (www.healthywater.com)

Foods and Herbs That Inhibit *H Pylori*

General

Kockar, C *et al*. 2001. *Helicobacter pylori* eradication with beta-carotene, ascorbic acid and allicin. *Acta Medica*. 44(3):97-100.

C. Romero *et al. In vitro* activity of olive oil polyphenols against *Helicobacter pylori. J Agric Food Chem*: 55: 680-686.

D'Addario C. *et al.* Bactericidal Activity of Grape, Soy Flour, Tomato and Bramble Leaf Extracts to *Helicobacter pylori. Helicobacter* 2007 (P126); 12: 379-476.

O'Mahony, R *et al.* Bactericidal & Anti-adhesive Properties of Spices Against *Helicobacter pylori. Helicobacter* 2004 (A11.03); 9: 487-604.

Stoicova, C. 2008. Green Tea Inhibits *Helicobacter* Growth *in vivo* and *in vitro. Int J Antimicrob Agents.*

Woeller, K. 2006. *Resolving Chronic Stress Related Disorders*. Biohealth Diagnostics DVD set.

Murray, MT. *The Healing Power of Herbs*. Rocklin, CA. Prima Publishing; 1995:165.

Fukai T., Maruma A., Kaitou K., Kanada T., Terada S., Nomura T., Anti-*Helicobater* flavonoids from Licorice extrat. *Life Sciences*. 2002; 1449-1463.

Berries

Chatterjee, A. *et al.* 2004. Inhibition of *Helicobacter pylori* in vitro by various berry extracts, with enhanced susceptibility to Clarithromycin. *Journal Molecular and Cellular Biochemistry*, 265:1-2, 19-26.

Matshushima *et al.* The Growth Inhibitory Effects of Cranberry Extract on *Helicobacter pylori* – In Vitro analysis. *Helicobacter* 2005 (A01.15); 10: 458-556.

Lin YT *et al.* Inhibition of *Helicobacter pylori* and associated urease by oregano and cranberry phytochemical synergies. *App Env Microb*. 2005; 71(12): 8558-64.

Sulforaphane

Fahey, J *et al.* 2002. Sulforaphane inhibits extracellular, intracellular, and anti-biotic resistant strains of *Helicobacter pylori* and prevents benzo[a]pyrene-induced stomach tumours. *PNAS*: 99:11, 7610-7615.

Cabbage Juice / Vitamin U

Cheney G. Rapid healing of peptic ulcers in patients receiving fresh cabbage juice. *Calif Med*. 1949 Jan; 70(1):10–15.

Cheney G. Vitamin U therapy of peptic ulcer. *Calif Med*. 1952 Oct; 77(4):248–252.

Cheney G. The nature of the antipepticulcer dietary factor. *Stanford Med Bull*. 1950 Aug; 8(3):144–161.

Cheney, G. Vitamin U concentrate therapy of peptic ulcer. Am J Gastroenterol. 1954 Mar; 21(3):230–250.

Tsimmerman, IaS, Golovanova, ES. Clinical effect and an analysis of the mechanism of action of vitamin U (S-methylmethioninesulfonium chloride) in peptic ulcer of the stomach and duodenum. *Ter Arkh*. 1976; 48(3):29-35. Russian.

Mastic Gum

Pataschos S, Magiatis P, Mitakou S, et al. In vitro and in vitro activities of Chios mastic gum extracts and constituents against Helicobacter pylori. *Antimicrob Agents Chemother*. 2007. Feb; 51 (2):551-9. Epub 2006 Nov 20.

Marone P, Bono L, Leone E. Bacterial activity of Pistacia leticus mustic gum against Helicobacter pylori. *J Chemother*. 2001 Dec; 13(6):611-4.

Huwez FU, Thirlwell D, Cockayne A. Mustic gum kills Helicobacter pylori. *N Engl J Med*. 1998; Dec 24; 339(26):1946.

Al-Habbal MJ, Al Habbal Z, Huwez FU. A double-blind controlled clinical trial of mastic and placebo in the treatment of duodenal ulcer. *Clin Exp Pharmacol Physiol* 1984; 11:541-544.

Bouic, P 2006. BioActivity Screening Services. Matula Tea Technical and Reference Manual. Synexa Life Sciences.

Vitamin C

Zhang HM et al. 1997. Vitamin C inhibits the growth of a bacterial risk factor for gastric carcinoma: Helicobacter. *Cancer* 80:1897-1903.

Jarosz M. 1998. Effects of high dose vitamin C treatment on Helicobacter pylori infection and total vitamin C concentration in gastric juice. *Eur J Cancer Prev* 7:449-454.

Zinc-L-Carnosine

Odashima M. Zink L-carnosine protects colonic muosal injury through induction of heat stock protein 72 abd suppression of NF-kappaB activation. *Life Sci*. 2006 Nov 10; 79(24):2245-50.

Mahmood A, Fitzgerald AJ. Zinc carnosine, a health food supplement that stabilizes small bowel integrity and stimulates gut repair process. *Gut*. 2007 Feb; 56(2):168-75.

Mikami K, Otaka M, Watanabe D. Zink L-carnosine protects against mucosal injury in portal hypertensive gastropathy through induction of heat stock protein 72. *J Gastroenterol Hepatol.* 2006. Nov; 21(11):1669-74.

Mishkin S. Intriguing gastrointestinal properties of bismuth: a folk remedy brought into the realm of clinical and investigative medicine. *Can J Gastroenterol* 1998; 12:569-570.

Lactoferrin

Imoto, I *et al.* Suppressive Effect of Bovine Lactoferrin against Helicobacter pylori. *Helicobacter* 2004 (A11.27); 9: 487-604.

Di Mario, F. Efficacy of bovine lactoferrin for Helicobacter pylori eradication: Results of a multicenter study. *Helicobacter* 2004 (A11.03); 9: 487-604.

Aragona, G *et al.* Lactoferrin in a 1-Week Triple Therapy for Eradication of H pylori. *Helicobacter.* 2003 (A16.06); 8: 339-493.

***Lactobacilli* and Probiotics**

Jarosz, M. Evaluation of the Vitamin C and Probiotic Use in *Helicobacter pylori* Infection Eradication Treatment. *Helicobacter.* 2003 (A13.08); 8: 339-493.

Johnson C, Jonsson H & Roos, S. Anti-*Helicobacter* pylori Activity Among Lactic Acid Bacteria Isolated from Gastric Biopsies and Strains of *Lactobacillus reuteri. Helicobacter.* 2003 (A16.33); 8: 339-493.

Bajenov *et al.* Anti-*Helicobacter* pylori activity of *Lactobacillus*, isolated from gastric juice and saliva. *Helicobacter.* 2003 (A15.03); 8: 339-493.

Connolly E *et al.* Dietary Supplementation with the Probiotic *Lactobacillus reuteri* (ATCC 55730) Leads to Colonisation of the Human Stomach and Duodenum. *Helicobacter.* 2003 (A04:27); 8: 339-493.

Myllyluoma, E *et al.* Effects of Probiotic Mixture in *Helicobacter pylori* Eradication therapy. *Helicobacter.* 2003 (A15.02); 8: 339-493.

Diaz-Reganon Vilches, J *et al.* 2005. Probiotics against *Helicobacter pylori*. Is there any effect? *Helicobacter.* 2005 (A01.14); 10: 458-556.

Haukioja A *et al.* 2005. Inhibition of *Helicobacter pylori* by Probiotic and Dairy Lactobacillus Strains. *Helicobacter.* 2005 (A01.09); 10: 458-556.

Moreno *et al.* Effect of probiotic lactic acid bacteria isolated from foods against *Helicobacter pylori. Helicobacter.* 2005 (A01.011); 10: 458-556.

Bielanski W *et al.* Improvement of anti-*Helicobacter pylori* therapy by the use of commercially available probiotics. *Helicobacter* 2002; 7: A98.

Brito *et al.* Evaluation of the inhibitory activity of *Lactobacillus* species from table olives against *Helicobacter pylori. Helicobacter* 2007 (P091); 12: 379-476.

Saccharomyces boulardii

Buts JP *et al*. Stimulation of Secretory IgA and Seretory Component of Immunoglobulins in Small Intestine of Rats Treated with *Saccharomyces boulardii*. *Dig Dis Sci* 35; 2:251-256.

Buts JP et al. *Saccharomyces boulardii* for *Clostridium difficile* Disease – Associated enteropathies in Infants. *J Pedriat Gastroenterol Nutr*. 1993. 16:419-425.

Ducluzeau, R and Bensaada M. Comparative Effect of a Single or Continuous Administration of *S boulardii* on the Establishment of Various Strains of *Candida* in the Digestive Tract of Gnotobiotic Mice. *Ann Microbiol*. 1982; 1338:491-501.

www.gastrohep.com/news/news.asp?id=2031

Parasite and Yeast/Fungal Overgrowth Questionnaire

As you've seen in this book, parasites and fungal overgrowth can cause many symptoms, often seemingly unrelated to the digestive tract. They are sadly underestimated by doctors and the medical system.

Please circle the number on the right hand side if you answer 'YES' to a question.

	Points
1. Have you ever taken antibiotics?	**1**
2. Have you taken birth control pills for six months or more?	**2**
3. Do you currently have athlete's foot, nail fungus, jock itch or skin conditions such as psoriasis, urticarial or dermatitis?	**1**
4. Do you have food sensitivities or allergies?	**2**
5. Do you have chemical or environmental sensitivities (for example, perfumes, petrol fumes, car exhausts, cleaning products)?	**2**
6. Do you crave sugar, sweets, starches or alcohol?	**2**
7. Do you crave bread, pasta, baked goods or do you "always want more" when you eat them?	**2**
8. Do you feel low on energy or drained?	**1**
9. Do you experience burping, belching or bloating?	**2**
10. Do you find it hard to focus or concentrate on tasks?	**2**
11. Do you experience moodiness, emotional sensitivity or difficulty dealing with stress?	**2**
12. Do you have muscle aches, joint pain and stiffness?	**1**

13. Do you experience an itchy nose, itchy   **2**
eyes or an itchy rectum?

14. Do you experience constipation and/or diarrhea?   **2**

15. Have you lost weight inexplicably, or do you   **2**
have an abnormally high or low appetite?

16. Do you have a swollen or distended belly?   **2**

17. Do you have close contact with pets or   **2**
other animals?

18. Do you have dark circles under your eyes?   **2**

19. Do you have adult acne?   **1**

20. Do you experience a worsening of symptoms   **1**
at night?

Now, add your total points: ———

What conclusions can you derive from your results:

6-10 Points: you certainly have signs of parasites and/or yeast and fungal overgrowth and may benefit from stool testing and / or a parasite cleanse.

11+ Points: you almost certainly have a parasitic and/or yeast overgrowth. You should consider speaking to a specialist, running comprehensive stool testing or running thorough yeast, fungal and parasite cleanses.

Please do not hesitate to contact us if you think we can help.

Email **Office@HPExperts.com**, call **0800 310 21 21** or see **www.H-Pylori-Symptoms.com/consultation** for information on our consultancy, lab testing and digestive balancing services.

Adrenal Stress/Fatigue Questionnaire

Assign a number between 0 and 5.

0 = Not true   3 = Somewhat true   5 = Very true

Once you have completed the questionnaire calculate your total and locate the range you fall under.

1. I experience problems falling asleep.	0 3 5	
2. I experience problems staying asleep.	0 3 5	
3. I frequently experience a second wind (high energy) late at night.	0 3 5	
4. I have energy highs and lows throughout the day.	0 3 5	
5. I feel tired all the time.	0 3 5	
6. I need caffeine (coffee, tea, cola, etc) to get going in the morning.	0 3 5	
7. I usually go to bed after 10pm.	0 3 5	
8. I frequently get less than 8 hours of sleep per night.	0 3 5	
9. I am easily fatigued.	0 3 5	
10. Things I used to enjoy seem like a chore lately.	0 3 5	
11. My sex drive is lower than it used to be.	0 3 5	
12. I suffer from depression, or have recently been experiencing feelings of depression such as sadness, or loss of motivation.	0 3 5	
13. If I skip meals I feel low energy or foggy and disoriented.	0 3 5	
14. My ability to handle stress has decreased.	0 3 5	
15. I find that I am easily irritated or upset.	0 3 5	

16. I have had one or more stressful major life events. (ie: divorce, death of a loved one, job loss, new baby, new job)   **0 3 5**

17. I tend to overwork with little time for play or relaxation for extended periods of time.   **0 3 5**

18. I crave sweets.   **0 3 5**

19. I frequently skip meals or eat sporadically.   **0 3 5**

20. I am experiencing increased physical complaints such as muscle aches, headaches, or more frequent illnesses.   **0 3 5**

Now, add your total points: _____

Scoring Your Adrenal Stress Profile:

It is important to note that this is not a diagnostic test and should not be used to diagnose any medical conditions. It is simply a tool to help assess your likely level of adrenal burnout.

0 – 30   **You likely are in good health.**

30 – 40   **You likely are under some stress.**

40 - 50   **You likely are a candidate for adrenal burnout.**

50 – 60   **You likely are in adrenal burnout.**

60 +   **You may be in severe adrenal burnout.**

If you have scored 40 or higher you are in adrenal burnout and will more than likely at some point experience the symptoms such as fatigue, weight gain, insomnia, irritability, and mood swings.